E50

12.50

XRAY LIBRARY
ROBERT L. MEALS D.O.,

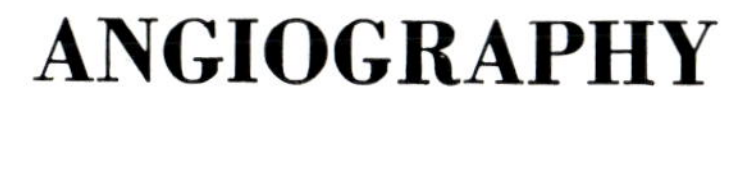

ANGIOGRAPHY

ANGIOGRAPHY

Techniques and Procedures

By

JOSEPH E. WHITLEY, M. D.
Professor of Radiology

and

NANCY O'NEIL WHITLEY, M. D.
Assistant Professor of Radiology

The Bowman Gray School of Medicine
of Wake Forest University
Winston-Salem, North Carolina, U.S.A.

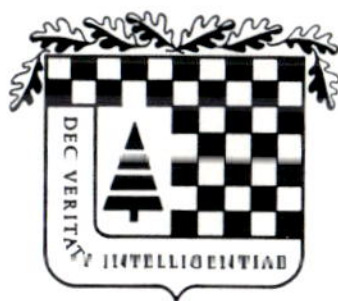

WARREN H. GREEN, INC.
St. Louis, Missouri, U.S.A.

Published by

WARREN H. GREEN, INC.
10 South Brentwood Blvd.
St. Louis, Missouri 63105, U.S.A.

All rights reserved.

© *1971 by WARREN H. GREEN, INC.*

Library of Congress Catalog Card No. 76-111804

Printed in the United States of America
1-A (181)

To

the memory of James Picker,
Founder of the James Picker Foundation

Acknowledgements

THE AUTHORS GRATEFULLY ACKNOWLEDGE the art work of Mr. George Lynch and Mrs. Jane Elolf, the photography of Mr. Jack Dent, the daily efforts of my Chief Technologist, Mr. Harold Cooke, and the assistance in manuscript preparation of Mrs. Edna Snow, and Dr. William F. Harriss.

Contents

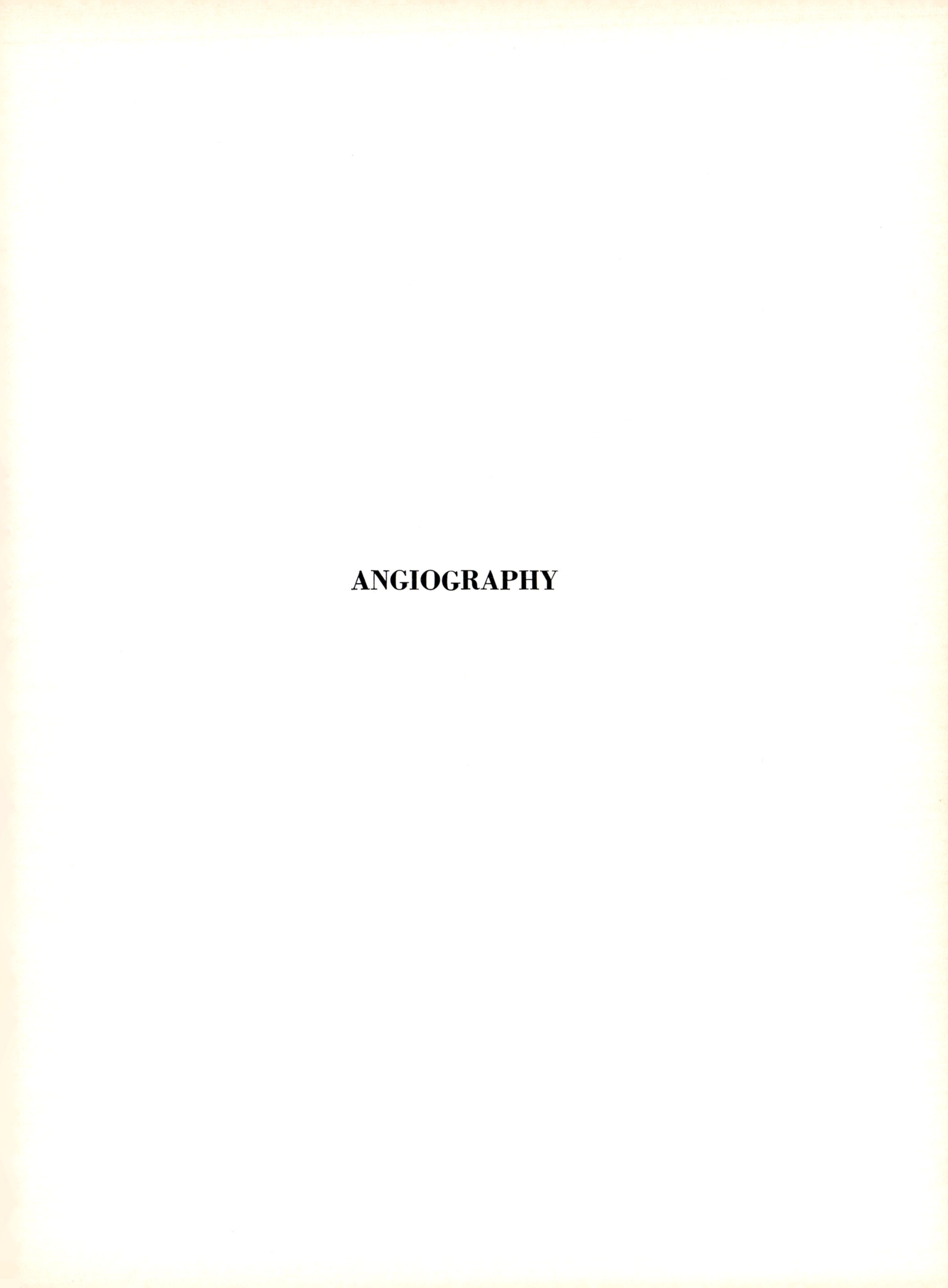

ANGIOGRAPHY

1

Introduction

GONE ARE THE DAYS when angiography was learned journeyman-style by observing or assisting in a few "sticks" or "caths" and when procedures were limited, apparatus primitive and results often questionable. The increase in scope and sophistication of these procedures now requires manual dexterity enhanced by thorough knowledge of principles and considerable self-catechism concerning the dangers and the manifold possibilities.

The purpose of the book is to furnish a first estimate of technique, practical details and some thoughts that should run through the minds of the individuals of an angiographic team approaching a study. A pragmatic approach to the phsical requirements of the room, machines, and materials involved is put forth not as exclusive dogma, but a simple workable way.

The techniques and philosophy presented have largely been adapted from work of others and evolved by a group of special procedure technologists and physicians from the Departments of Radiology, Medicine, Neurology and Surgery at The Bowman Gray School of Medicine. I hope it will be added to and revised often by anyone naive enough to adopt it. The doses, etc., are designed for that mythical 70 Kg adult in blank physiologic state and are not magic. Applied without thought, they will frequently result in mediocrity and could be dangerous.

All "good" angiography is a term relative to time, place, clinical indications and degree of emergency. That a specialized medical physician, a radiologist and a surgeon skilled in the particular area are all usually needed is obvious. This is as true in the "countryside" as the university hospital. Studies should not be done without some physician available to care for any possible complication of, and usually perform definite surgery for any possible outcome. "Good" angiography can and should be more widely practiced than it is today.

Future progress in the field of angiography will come from physicians of many backgrounds but principally those who not only specialize in "special procedures," but sub-specialize in a single or small group of diseases, techniques of examination, as well as the anatomy, physiology and pathology of his focused interests. However, these individuals will not exist in a vacuum, for to contribute they must relate to others with medical, surgical, and radiologic knowledge, interest and skills in their allied areas.

A special procedure can be no better than the technologists who contribute so significantly to it. The complexity and irascibility of the machines (and physicians) with which they work, and the responsibility for patient welfare and the diagnostic result which they share, place them in a unique minority of paramedical personnel along with anesthetists and intensive care nurses. Their willingness to accept responsibility, perform daily under stress, their personal honesty and their ability deserve the physician's respect. The angiographer who is abusive of a capable technologist is usually angry at his own inadequacies and should be tolerated only for the sake of his patient. Such a person does nothing to stabilize a team and should find a more comfortable area of work for himself, referring patients for the studies to someone with more adequate skill and/or personality.

This brief outline of radiographic technique is written for physicians with some radiologic background who are in training or trained and forming or joining a team to perform "special procedures." It is not meant to challenge the more complex clinical and research techniques of the many excellent general and specialized angiographic teams which exist in medical centers scattered throughout the world.

The references included rarely list the "first" publication on the subject. They were largely selected from the recent literature. This book is meant to be written in, so that the references can be added to and updated by the reader, and the technical details altered to fit the machines and tastes of the group employing them.

2

Physical Requirements

As recently as 1964, a 296 page book on hospital design (8) failed to mention special diagnostic radiology. The only space recommendation in regard to diagnostic radiology was "300 to 350 assignable square feet of net floor space per x-ray technologist (add 50 per cent for corridors, stairs, elevators, toilets, shafts, etc.)." Other more recent texts (4) identify the term and one is quite valuable (6). This illustrates the lack of, or lag in, communication between physicians and architects which has caused problems for all concerned in the past.

THE ROOM

To optimally plan even one room is to plan: (1) a scrub area or room; (2) a room for loading the film for the changer; (3) a control and generator room (or two separate rooms for this purpose); (4) a film viewing area; (5) the procedure room itself; (6) plus a physiologic monitoring room or alcove if pressures, oxygens, etc. are to be performed. To superimpose these on a typical 300 net footage per technologist plan is difficult and many compromises ensue. In some departments, even the minimum ceiling height of nine and one-half feet may be difficult to find. Three hundred to 350 square feet may be adequate for a procedure room itself but an equal or larger area for the supporting functions outlined above, plus 50 per cent of the whole for "corridors, stairs, etc." is necessary.

In planning new construction where there will be patient demand sufficient to allow multiple rooms for special procedures, there is every advantage in planning each room to be equipped and adapted to one or a small number of closely allied procedures. The idea of multiple multipurpose rooms as a desirable arrangement for a large department is dead in special procedures as well as routine diagnosis. Where economically feasible, specialized physicians working with specialized radiologic technologists and specialized equipment offer the best, most efficient patient care.

Ideally, whether it is a single special procedure room or an elaborate multiroom complex, it should be somewhat isolated from routine radiography because of patient and medical traffic. A location readily available to the emergency entrance of the hospital (ambulance entry), the surgical area, and routine diagnosis is ideal. When compromises as to location have to be made, proximity to the routine diagnostic radiology area is probably most important.

If a number of special procedure rooms are planned, they usually should be grouped together. This affords the efficiency of sharing a proper scrub room and dressing and locker areas; a central supply room for sterile supplies; accessory storage; dark room; and most impotant, a core of specially trained technologists. Where economy requires it, this arrangement allows paired large generators to be shared by contiguous procedure rooms. A cul de sac or spur corridor is ideal with no through traffic and limited admittance into what should be a clean area. This design has the shortcoming of being difficult to expand when the need arises.

What do you buy for a single multipurpose room in a hospital unable to support multiple specialized rooms? The most likely answer is a single plane TV with cine, a single or preferably biplane film changer, and an "island" table with a moving top.

Television fluoroscopy is a practical necessity for modern day arteriography. When a group of special procedure rooms is planned, there is a definite advantage to planning a broadcast-type TV control room with a high quality sync (synchronization) generator and back-up sync generator, rather than the multiple cheap industrial sync generators which would be routinely furnished by a commercial x-ray company. This offers the possibility of sharing one or more centrally placed quality tape recorders with the signals from all rooms being compatible. Such a system was designed and developed by Dr. James F. Martin, Mr. Don Polley and Mr. Harold Cooke, and has been in operation at this institution since 1961. Broadcast-type signal wave form monitors also help keep the cameras in optimum adjustment.

Ceiling or wall mounting the TV monitor and the physiologic monitoring oscilloscope is usually a convenience and a space saver. Some angiographic tables offer plug plates in their bases for connecting EKG, injector, changer, and strain guage via subfloor conduits to appropriate curcuits. Such a modification is possible in most machines and the conduit system is worth its cost in freeing the procedure room from the maze of wires which otherwise stretch across it.

With TV fluoroscopy, room lighting should be reheostat controlled. At present, incandescent lighting is more trouble-free than the newer intensity adjustable fluorescents. A ceiling or wall mounted operating room type spot light is a great convenience.

The problem of grounding of all conductors which come in contact with the patient is a real one. An adequate common ground should be planned for special procedure rooms. The water pipe may not be useable due to its conductivity or multiple usage. Newer electromechanical injectors are frequently built to electrically isolate the syringe from its power sources. The problem of explosive anesthetics in a special radiographic procedure room is probably best solved by using only their non-explosive alternates when anesthesia is necessitated.

EQUIPMENT

Generators. The argument as to full-wave rectified versus three phase generators has finally been settled, at least for special procedures. Three phase generators, big ones, are the winners. The reason is the radiation absorption characteristics of iodine which, in the form of organic iodides, is today's contrast medium for angiography. To obtain a serialogram with optimum iodine contrast, quick high milliamperage orthovoltage exprosures are required. Due to variations in techniques of machine calibration, beam filtration, and screen-film-developer combinations, it is not possible to specify what the proper maximum Kv is. It rarely exceeds 80 to 90 Kv.

Excellent angiography can be done with a good 500 milliampere, full-wave rectified generator in the majority of clinical situations and the majority of patients. The clinical reason for the 1000, 1250 milliampere and larger three phase genrators is the huge patient and the patient who cannot or will not cooperate. Cine and TV techniques neither need nor profit by huge generators.

Almost equal in importance with the size and type of generator is the adequacy of the power supply. The modern big generators have power requirements in the order of 125 to 165 KvA each and despite the built-in voltage compensation circuits they are quite sensitive to instantaneous voltage fluctuation. A separate transformer for a diagnostic radiology department is a necessity, and in large departments more than one may be needed. A circuit to prevent simultaneous exposure in the department has recently been described (5).

Image Amplifiers. Six and seven inch image amplifiers offer maximum amplification and are adequate in field size. Nine inch and six-nine combinations are thought more comfortable by some angiographers. It has been demonstrated that, for clinical purposes, careful cine technique can replace large film angiograms in many anatomic areas. This approach seems most useful in relatively small anatomic areas as the heart, although by moving the camera and following the bolus of medium, even femoral arteriography has been successfully performed (3, 7). Television taping has similarly been used for venography. TV and cine have their place in angiography; however, for most, if not all, of the procedures described in this text, large serialography is the technique of choice. In some examinations this is due to the extreme definition of small vessels needed, and in others due to large dimension of the field of interest.

Changers. The choice of changers is wide and growing wider. They can be divided into:

Orthodox Version	*Specialty Version*
Metal cassette changers	Long film (leg) changer
Vacumm cassette changers	
Roll film changers	"See through" changer[1]
Cut film changers	"See through" changer"

Metal cassette changers have the problem of being limited in rapidity of filming and the number of films which can be obtained. Except for specialty types employing long films for examination of the legs, I cannot recommend them.

The vacuum cassette changer is an ingenious design and appears to have long term wearing ability. The roll film design has proven itself; however, it has the minor problems of difficulty in adjusting screen contact and film waste due to leader, and reloading "early" to be sure of enough film for the next series. The "see through" changers incorporating an image amplifier as the backing for the film stage is the newest breakthrough and should speed and simplify some examinations. The present maximum filming rate of these devices, two per second, will obviously limit the range of examinations for which it can be used.

The classic cut film changer design is my personal favorite and has passed the test of long stability in the field. It is intolerant of high humidity and requires meticulous maintenance.

Tubes, Filters and Collimators. High speed rotation and small focal spot tubes are of great advantage in cine and serialograms. An automatically adjusting filter to vary the filtration of a beam with the kilovoltage to be imposed on the tube would be ideal, but not commercially available. Manually adjustable filters are commercially available. With specialized machines performing only one or a limited number of examinations, a properly selected fixed filter is adequate. I personally employ a 0.05 millimeter copper with two millimeters of aluminum below it for most angiography. For long leg changers, wedge filters are a necessity.

Precise collimators are essential and neither the circular aperture nor the rectangular aperture models are ideal for everything. There is a single combination round-rectangular model on the market which is incorporated on a specialized neuroradiologic unit. The rectangular is probably the best choice for general angiography; however, the addition of irregular diaphragms and extension cones is useful in certain examinations. For maximum detail in a limited area, there is still no substitute for the extension cone.

Tables. The typical GI table with the tube below and the image amplifier attached above with an arm is not satisfactory for special procedures. The structures connecting the arm to the table make working on that side of the table difficult. An island table with a four-way floating table top and the tube above or below is much nearer to the ideal. The problem then resolves itself into which goes under the table, the image tube or the x-ray tube. The advent of the see-through changer with the potential of checking catheter position and filming instantaneously may establish a tube above preference, providing a convenient method of positively aligning the x-ray beam and the amplifier is developed.

ACCESSORY EQUIPMENT

Due to the potential problems of patients undergoing special procedures, a complete set of resuscitation equipment and drugs should be in the room (2). An EKG monitoring device is essential in certain catheterization procedures in and around the heart and desirable in almost all special radiologic procedures. A D.C. defibrillator should be available to the angiography laboratory and physically in it during selected cases. A strain gauge pressure transducer, monitor and recorder is a useful device in many types of procedures. Piping in oxygen and suction from a central system into a special procedure room, just as in an intensive care unit, is worthwhile.

REFERENCES

1. Amplatz, K.: New rapid roll-film changer. Radiology, 90:130-134, Jan. 1968.
2. Barnhard, H. J., and Barnhard, F. M.: The emergency treatment of reactions to contrast media: updated 1968. Radiology, 91:74-84, July 1968.
3. Gyepes, M. T., and Abrams, H. L.: Peripheral cine arteriography. Radiology, 88:736-739, April 1967.
4. Hudenburg, R.: *Planning the Community Hospital.* New York, McGraw-Hill, 1967.
5. McGinnis, K. D., Smith, L. A., and Mills, G. L.: Analysis of simultaneous radiographic exposures. Radiology, 92:1481-1484, June 1969.
6. Morgan, R. H., and others: Rooms for Special Diagnostic Procedures. In: *Planning Guide for Radiologic Installations,* 2nd ed., edited by W. G. Scott. Baltimore, Williams & Wilkins, 1966, ch. 7, pp. 44-59.
7. Skinner, G. B.: The use of cinefluorography in peripheral arteriography. Amer. J. Roentgenol., 95: 745-750, Nov. 1965.
8. Wheeler, E. Todd: *Hospital Design and Function.* New York, McGraw-Hill, 1964.

3

METHODS AND MATERIALS

THERE ARE TWO METHODS of entering the vascular system: puncturing the vessel percutaneously, and surgically isolating a vessel and performing a formal arteriotomy. In adults with good femoral pulses and no history of claudication, the percutaneous method to gain entry to the aorta via the distal route is the most popular technique. In techniques where it is necessary or desirable to primarily introduce a catheter into the proximal aorta, there is disagreement as to the preferred method of entry. Logically, the training and experience of the operator will have much to do with his choice of technique. No one can argue with the technique of a successful angiographer so long as his complication rate is reasonable and comparable with other options.

Direct puncture of a vessel and the injection of contrast medium without the introduction of a catheter often offers simplicity and speed in accessible vessels. The disadvantages are the inability to change the site of injection or selectively inject vessels other than the one entered. The problem of arterial damage due to motion of a sharp, rigid needle during final positioning and while the films are checked, can be eliminated with a sheath needle (removing the needle and leaving the flexible sheath). Immobilizing the needle with some device (flats and sterile adhesive or an appropriate metal prop (15) can also help prevent injury. Another potentially preventable problem of this technique is the inadvertent subselective injection and partial extravasation. These problems can usually be averted by visualizing a small test injection either with Polaroid or TV visualization.

The introduction of a guide wire and/or a catheter(17) offers the advantage of selection of the site of injection, and pressure analysis and sampling at a distance from the puncture site. The additional disadvantages of this technique over direct puncture alone consist of more time and materials and the possibility of vascular injury remote to the site of entry. Using long sheath needles and a guide wire manipulating device, selective catheterization has been performed by the translumbar aortic technique (1,19).

Formal surgical arteriotomy usually requires more time, skill and materials. There is usually some patient discomfort due to occlusion of the distal artery during the procedure. In smaller arteries, arterial spasm occasionally makes catheter manipulation difficult and lastly is the possible deformity of the vessel lumen caused by closure.

MATERIALS

Needles. An organization of the many styles of needles employed for angiography is listed in Table A. No attempt will be made to list every eponym as the list would be so long as to be worthless.

The venopuncture needle is the least expensive and has the sharpest bevel of the usual needles employed. It is very satisfactory for percutaneous vein puncture without making any skin nick. Its sharpness is a potential disadvantage with arterial puncture making wall damage and even transection of an entire vessel possible.

The arteriographic needles such as the Cournand possess a less steep bevel, an obturator and frequently a specialized flange for grasping the needle during puncture. Each of these features offers an advantage in arterial puncture. Each type of flange has its following and much has to do with the individual's training. The needles with a secondary blunt obturator longer than the cannula offer the possibility of more safety in threading a vessel once puncture has been accomplished.

The Seldinger style needle has a sharp protruding obturator with a low profile bevel and small central stylet. It is designed to be inserted assembled. The stylet is removed and the pulsatile flow of arterial blood indentifies the lumen of the vessel as the needle is withdrawn. The sharp obturator is removed and the shorter blunt needle then remains completely within the vessel lumen. The obturator and stylet are frequently removed as a unit prior to withdrawal of the needle in an adult femoral puncture. The localizing feature of the stepwise removal of stylet and then obturator can be important in smaller vessels.

Most modern arteriographic needles have blunt tip with a sharp protruding obturator and matching protruding blunt obturator. A wire guide type obturator has been designed (18).

The sheath needles are a variation on the arteriographic design with a flexible plastic sheath fitted over the needle slightly shorter than the bevel. It is inserted and when the lumen is encountered, the needle is withdrawn and the sheath remains and can be threaded into the vessel. Once the needle has been removed, it should not be re-inserted into the sheath except under direct vision as the needle can cut the plastic sheath.

TABLE A

Needles

Venopuncture (steep bevel) standard and thin-walled.

Sharp arteriographic (less steep bevel) with matching obturators with or without secondary protruding blunt obturator.

Seldinger needle, blunt needle with sharp protruding obturator with matching central style.

Blunt arteriolgraphic needle with sharp protruding obturator and matching protruding blunt obturators.

Sheath needle with matching flexible plastic sheath fitted over it which is to remain after the needle is withdrawn.

Catheters. If a catheter is to be introduced, a decision as to type must be made. The classic vascular (cardiac) catheters were an adaptation of ureteral catheters. They were a woven fabric tubing which was coated with appropriate plastic materials. The original size of the lumen relative to the external diameter made the instrument more suitable for pressure and sampling than injection. A relatively thin-walled, more supple design was forthcoming. In addition to the simple end opening, a closed end tube with side openings was made to prevent recoil with pressure injection. The ends of these devices are shaped either by autoclaving with a removeable curved wire stylet in the distal two to three inches (in the end-opening variety), or by means of an external splint (in the closed-end types). They are designed to be re-used and sterilized with autoclaving. The cardiac catheter was not designed to be used percutaneously and does not bevel at its tip; however, employing an appropriate mylar sheath over a percutaneous catheter, this type of catheter can be introduced. With exposure to body temperature, it becomes more flexible and loses its shaping. It can be molded in the vascular system by lodging it in an appropriate shape for a few minutes and "setting it" with a flush of any cold (room temperature) liquid.

The classic percutaneous catheter material is Ödman's barium-loaded polyethylene (13), which is ductile and malleable in 75° C hot water, steam or air. It allows the operator to readily form a tip design and catheter shape and change design to fit the anatomic circumstances at the time of procedure. Because of the inconvenience of cold sterilization and the lack of excellent torque response, other materials have come on the market; however, the facility for rapid re-design of a catheter has not been surpassed.

Factory pre-formed catheters, as those made over the curve patterns, will accomplish more than ninety per cent of clinical angiography. These are available in sterile disposable form as are most of the catheter materials in Table B. Fabricated forming wires of most of the shapes employed are commercially available.

Another approach in placing catheters selectively in the vascular tree has been the design of a manipulating device which could predictably change the shape of a catheter. Many inventions of various degrees of complexity have been made and manufactured for sale. None of these devices is essential for angiography. Proving the superiority of one over another in the cases where "something extra" is desirable, is difficult due to the number of devices and techniques available. Some of these instruments are very ornery and complex relative to their small talents. But every father loves his child, and some of these instruments are lucky to have a dad with residents who are forced to master the techniques of working with the little wonder.

Of the crop, the Cook Catheter Tip Deflector* and the Medi-Tech Selector™ catheter** seem to offer a reasonable supplement and an alternative to the classic technique of fashioning catheters to perform selectives in the difficult case and in subselective studies.

Injectors. The original was the hand and a syringe. This system is still excellent for test injections and situations where there is a low blood flow to

---

*Cook Inc., Bloomington, Indiana 47401.
William Cook, Europe A/S, DK 2730 Herlev, Denmark.

**Medi-Tech, Inc., Belmont, Mass. 02178.

be momentarily replaced. The lever was a logical extension to magnify muscle power and produce more rapid flow rates.

Compressed gas, spring and electric motored models are currently on the market. The most elegant models presently are electric motor driven and produced by Barber Coleman Company* (the Viamonte Hobbs) Medrad, Inc.† (the Heilman-Wholey) and the Cordis Corporation.‡

The feature of these injectors which sets them off from their predecessors is that they bring more sharply into focus the end result of dosage as a function of speed and injection time. Of course, the strength of the injectors and the bursting point of catheters remain finite. In the usual clinical situation, the optimum injection rate replaces the blood flow (cc/sec) of the vessel being examined. The Cordis model calculates the range of injection rates possible with the viscosity of the medium, and the length and lumen size of the catheter being employed. The operator then selects the pressure and time to correspond. With the Viamonte Hobbs, and the Heilman-Wholey "dose-rate" and time are set directly. Maximum injections rates per catheter and medium combination are stated on a chart of furnished maximum rate. Both offer the operator a check of the actual delivered dose in the time set by checking the calibrated syringe after an injection. With other injectors it is necessary to obtain or determine with a stop watch and the media employed, charts of pressure versus catheter length and lumen size for a logical approach to injector usage. With less complex and expensive injectors and such charts, good angiography is readily performed.

Contrast Media. The choice of intravascular contrast agents depends on its opacity, viscosity, lack of toxicity, and expense. The substitution of meglumine (methylglucamine) for most or all of the sodium of the earlier salts of the present day triiodized contrast compounds has resulted in greater patient comfort and less induced localized and systemic hyperosmolarity. The tolerance of individual end organs to various media remains under investigation, and close attention should be paid to the precautions of the drug inserts.

TABLE B

RADIOPAQUE CATHETER MATERIALS

	Poly-ethylene	*Poly-vinyl*	*Teflon*	*Polyurethane Encapsulated on Metal Braid* ¶
Friction of Usual Finish	Medium	Medium	Low	Medium
Curve Retention	Good	Good	Excellent §	Excellent
Kinking Tendency	Low	Low	Moderate	Very low
Torque Response	Fair ‖	Fair ‖	Good	Excellent
Resistance to Bursting Pressure	Moderate ‖	Moderate ‖	High	High
Effect of Temperature and Moisture of the Blood on Flexibility	Minimal increase	Moderate increase	None	None
Sterilization	Cold	Autoclave	Autoclave	Cold

* Barber Coleman Co., Rockport, Ill. 61101.
†Medrad, Inc., Allison Park, Pa. 15101.
‡Cordis Corporation, Miami, Florida 33127.
§When tempered in open flame, or 600°—1000° F heatgun(2).
‖Vary with wall thickness.
¶ Ducor®, Cordis Corporation, Miami, Florida 33137.

REFERENCES

1. Amplatz, K.: Translumbar catheterization of the abdominal aorta. Radiology, 81:927-931, Dec., 1963.
2. Amplatz, K., and Harner, R.: A new subclavian artery catheterization technique; preliminary report. Radiology, 78:963-966, June, 1962.
3. Baker, H. L.: A new approach to percutaneous subclavian angiography. Proc. Staff Meet. Mayo Clin., 35:169-174, March, 1960.
4. Boijsen, E., and Feinstein, G. L.: Arteriographic catheterization techniques. Amer. J. Roentgenol., 85:1037-1052, June, 1961.
5. Desilets, D. T., Hoffman, R. B., and Ruttenberg, H. D.: A new method of percutaneous catheterization. Amer. J. Roentgenol., 97:519-522, June, 1966.
6. Fischer, H. W.: Hemodynamic reactions to angiographic media; a survey and commentary. Radiology, 91:66-73, July 1968.
7. Fischer, H. W., Roller, G., and Hubbard, P. G.: An analysis of several factors influencing injection rate in angiography. Radiology, 83:396-404, Sept. 1964.
8. Hanafee, W.: Axillary artery approach to carotid, vertebral, abdominal aorta, and coronary angiography. Radiology, 81:559-567, Oct. 1963.
9. Klatte, E. C., Sloan, O. M., and Burko, H.: Selective teflon arteriographic catheters. Radiology, 90:1205-1206, June 1968.
10. Lindgren, E.: The technique of direct (percutaneous) cerebal angiography. Brit. J. Radiology, 20: 326, 1947.
11. Nebesar, R. A., Fleischli, D. J., Pollard, J. J., and Griscom, N. T.: Arteriography in infants and children: with emphasis on the Seldinger technique and abdominal diseases. Amer. J. Roentgenol., 106:81-91, May 1969.
12. Newton, T. H.: The axillary artery approach to arteriography of the aorta and its branches. Amer. J. Rotentgenol., 89:275-283, Feb. 1963.
13. Ödman, P.: The radiopaque polythene catheter. Acta Radiologica, 52:52-64, July 1959.
14. Olin, T.: Studies in Agiographic Technique. Hakan Ohlsson, Lund 1963.
15. Potts, D. G.: A needle and immobilization device for carotid angiography. Radiology, 92:1125-1126, Apr. 1969.
16. Roy, P.: Percutaneous catheterization via the axillary artery; a new approach to some technical roadblocks in selective arteriography. Amer. J. Roentgenol., 94:1-18, May 1965.
17. Seldinger, S. I.: Catheter replacement of the needle in percutaneous arteriography. Acta Radiologica, 39:368-376, 1953.
18. Sheldon, P.: Safer carotid angiography by percutaneous cannulation. Acta Radiol. Diagn., 5:517-522, 1966.
19. Stocks, L. O., Halpern, M., and Turner, A. F.: Complete translumbar aortography. Amer. J. Rotentgenol., 107:835-839, Dec. 1969.

4

COMPLICATIONS

THE INCIDENCE AND SEVERITY of complications vary with the vessel examined. Usually, coronary and cerebral arteriography have a higher complication rate; however, the skill of the angiography teams can almost suppress this difference (32). Examining a population of severely ill, or even terminal patients can produce dire results almost regardless of the type of examination or the skill of examiners. Table A summarizes some of the recent series of arteriographic complications. It is interesting in looking over this type of data to consider the complication rate of "no arteriography" which was encountered by Baum *et al.* (2). In a group of 1,600 patients in whom arteriography was performed, 9 serious and 5 fatal complications were encountered; versus 9 serious and 6 fatal "complications" which occurred in a group of patients within 48 hours of a scheduled arteriogram which was not performed.

Table B attempts to present a general outline of angiographic complications. The incidence of some of these complications will vary, not only with the skill of the angiographic team and with the severity of illness in the patient population, but with the judgment employed in choosing techniques to fit the individual patient and situation.

Neurogenic shock (near syncope, and rarely syncope) occur during angiography usually due to anxiety and the minimal trauma of skin anesthesia, or catheter manipulation. It is recognized by the patient's pallor, cold sweat or reporting a faint giddy sensation, and having thin rapid pulse. This stage may be followed by a full-blown vasovagal response with a slowing of the heart rate, fall in blood pressure and usually a loss of consciousness.

Prevention is ideal in this as other complications. Seeing the patient beforehand, allaying anxiety, an adequate preprocedural hypnotic drug and atropine, and proper local anesthesia may all be helpful. Despite all efforts, near syncope will occasionally happen. Recognition and prompt therapy is next best. Early, a deep whiff of aromatic spirits of ammonia and time will repair all. The EKG pattern should be checked for possible primary or secondary changes. Additional atropine given slowly intravenously and intravenous fluids may be indicated. A more rigorous approach with circulatory stimulants is rarely necessary.

Drug idiosyncrasy in arteriography is similar to that encountered in intravenous injection. Anaphylactoid shock is both difficult to predict and treat, particularly in the ill and elderly. A team trained in all out cardiopulmonary resuscitation with proper drugs and equipment is the only hope. Less severe reactions with histamine release can occasionally be predicted by the preliminary intravascular injection of one cc of medium. Routinely employing a prophylactic antihistamine has been suggested; however, we have not followed this recommendation except in occasional individuals with a history of reaction to a contrast medium. The treatment of drug reactions associated with histamine release is identical with that employed with intravenous pyelography.

Mechanical complications at the site of entry into the vascular system are among the more commonly encountered. It has been pointed out that many of the complications attributed to media in the literature are probably mechanical (1). When catheters or guide wires are employed, mechanical injury to vessels remote to the site of injury is possible. Prevention includes strict inspection of all materials to be placed in any vessel. Needles should be appropriately sharp with sleeves and obturators well fitted. Vessel dilators, catheters and guide wire should be free of defects. The patients' pulses in appropriate extremities should be recorded *prior* to beginning any arterial procedure.

The incidence of this type of complication will vary both with the dexterity of the primary operator and with his judgment employed in choice of technique and site of entry. Trauma distal to the site of entry caused by catheters and guide wires will also vary with skill and judgment. Care should be exercised in the selection of injection rates with end-opening catheters because of the jet phenomena and the local vascular collapse and damage which can be induced (12). Whipping can be a problem in high speed injections in end- and side-opening catheters (30). A sufficiently large catheter must be employed where large high speed injections must be delivered, particularly in the aortic arch.

Most mechanical complications during a procedure (i.e. undermining an atherosclerotic plaque, perforation of a vessel with a guide wire or catheter, and subintimal dissection) should usually be treated by observation and general supportive measures. Surgical intervention is only indicated by the patient's symptoms, obvious progression of signs, or both.

The patient's pulses should be examined and recorded as to presence and quality before arteriography, periodically during the procedure, and after removal of the needle and catheter. If an extremity pulse is lost during a procedure, a vasodilator, heparin and/or xylocaine may be administered locally into the involved artery via the needle or catheter prior to withdrawal.

Treatment for loss of a previously present pulse at the site of arteriotomy or arterial puncture varies with the artery involved. The pink, warm, asymptomatic extremity without a pulse can usually be watched expectantly for several hours. The cold, pale, painful extremity demands immediate surgical intervention. In either case, immediate systemic heparinization and a surgical consult are usually indicated. Spasm and thrombosis are unusual except in children and young women, and in small arteries. The prophylactic intra-arterial injection of procaine has been advocated to prevent spasm (17). We routinely employ this type of prohylaxis only in these high risk groups.

If signs of brachial plexus injury develop after an axillary artery puncture, immediate exploration of the axilla for hematoma of the neurovascular sheath should be carried out to minimize permanent neurologic deficit.

True chemotoxicity as defined by Lasser (25) is based on changes in blood elements, vascular endothelium and changes in other specific tissues. The three classic critical organs are the central nervous system, the heart, and the kidneys. The meglumine salt rather than the mixed meglumine and sodium, or the pure sodium salts of the modern contrast agents has been adopted for cerebral arteriography, because of the difference in the incidence of physiologic and pathologic abnormalities included. The initial clinical experience with one pure methylglucamine agent in coronary arteriography seems to indicate that a "mixed" salt with a small amount of sodium is advantageous. A clear superiority between the pure methylglucamine and the mixed (low sodium) salt has not been established for the kidney. The vasomotor effects of diatrizoates and iothalamates are less pronounced than with earlier media and are rarely a clinical problem.

Rouleaux formation of red blood cells and changes in platelet adhesiveness are caused by the methlglucamine media and may contribute to procedural and postprocedural thromboembolic complications (8). Low molecular weight dextran can reduce these phenomena (18). The intravenous administration of low molecular weight dextran (Macrodex®) (500 cc of 10%) prior to angiography has been suggested. Jacobsson noted this technique of using dextran may prolong bleeding time and thus may increase the incidence of pseudoaneurysm. Further investigation of the use of this agent particularly in high risk patients (i.e., those with clotting tendency or a history of transient ischemic episodes of the central nervous system) is warranted.

Stasis of media in a vessel, either due to catheter occlusion or intrinsic disease can, along with the accompanying anoxia, cause pain, spasm, and intimal inflammation. A classic example is phlebography of the lower extremities where, in varices, there is a high incidence of chemical phlebitis unless the media is "flushed out" with fluid after filming.

Despite the recent series demonstrating no prophylactic effect of 500 cc of 5% glucose prior to angiography (24), patients who are dehydrated, receive intravenous fluids when they arrive in our catheter laboratory as a nonspecific measure to limit chemotoxicity (6). The total dose of contrast is kept as small as possible, consistent with an optimal diagnostic study.

Thromboembolism and Hemorrhage. The problem of clotting in and around the catheter is complex, involving mechanical and chemotoxic factors. The smoothness, chemical and electrical characteristics of the catheter surface, the natural and induced clotting propensity of the patient's blood, the flow pattern of blood around the catheter, the area of catheter material exposed to the patient's blood, and the length of exposure of blood to the foreign surface are all factors.

The risk of thromboembolism is increased in children less than ten years of age and young females (probably due to their propensity to arterial spasm), severe atherosclerosis, and any condition leading to low cardiac output.

Jacobsson, working with radiopaque polythylene catheter materials has shown the caliber and length of the catheter to be of primary importance (19). Using oscillography to routinely monitor peripheral pulses is a sensitive method to detect subclinical thromboembolic phenomena. In the average patient, clots forming around the catheter which are milked off with removal, probably undergo lysis rapidly and are rarely a clinical problem. With low cardiac output, locally poor circulation or conceivably low circulating fibrinolysins, heparinization of the patient may be indicated. Symptomatic and asymptomatic impairment to arterial flow secondary to arterial catheterization in infants and young children may lead to inequality of leg growth, and the group represents a special problem (4).

The risk of local hemorrhage is increased by anticoagulants and hypertension. These two factors are relative contraindications to arteriography. According to the clinical indications for angiography, I know of no absolute contraindications. With warfarin therapy, vitamin K can sometimes be used to correct the prolonged prothrombin time. With severe hypertension, temporary intravenous antihypertensive therapy may be necessary for several hours after an arterial procedure to prevent hemorrhage.

TABLE A
COMPLICATIONS

Series	*Number*	*Technique*	*Fatal*	*Serious Nonfatal*	*Minor*
McAfee** 1957[28]	13,206	Translumbar 12,832	0.28	0.74	....
		Catheter 375			
Szilagyi* 1962[31]	2,399	Translumbar	0.04	0.46	....
Leadbetter*** 1962[26]	7,683	Translumbar	0	....	....
Lang** 1963[22]	14,642	Translumbar 3,240	0.03	0.34	3.6
		Seldinger 11,402	0.06	0.71	2.85
Bernstein** 1963[7]	1,339	Intravenous	0.15	0.22	2.1
Beall* 1964[5]	4,613	Translumbar	0.17	....	....
		"last 1388"	0.07	....	....
Halpern 1964[14]	1,000	Seldinger (femoral)	0	2.4	....
Taveras & Wood* 1964[32]	2,000	Cerebral	0	2	....
Allen et al* 1965[1]	538	Cerebral	0.19	3.7	....
Lodin & Ottander* 1966[27]	534	Carotid puncture	....	6	....
Hemley *et al*** 1967[16]	2,500	Intravenous aortography	0	....	....
Mortensen* 1967[29]	1,466	Direct puncture	0.14	1.2	10
	960	Cerebral	0.21	1.1	10.7
	158	Translumbar	0	0.6	4.4
	148	Femoral	0	1.4	10.8
	120	Radial	0	0	2.5
	46	Subclavian	0	0	13
	36	Brachial	0	8.9	33
	1,008	Cut-down	0.1	1.1	6.2
	560	External iliac	0	0.6	2.5
	308	Left subclavian	0.32	....	4
	140	Brachial	0	7.1	24.7
	719	Seldinger (femoral)	0.13	4.3	14.3
Haut & Amplatz* 1968[15]	1,000	Seldinger	0	1.8	..
	242	Translumbar	0	0.8	....
Hass *et al*** 1968	4,748	All	0.7	....	....

*Institutional source.

**Institutional and collected.

***Including 1,400 cases from Beall's series

TABLE B

1. Near syncope, syncope
2. Drug idiosyncracy, hypersensitivity:
    - Urticaria
    - Angioneurotic edema
    - Laryngeal edema
    - Rhinorrhea
    - Lacrimation
    - Sneezing
    - Pruritis
    - Laryngeal spasm
    - Bronchospasm
    - Anaphylactoid shock
3. Mechanical
4. True Chemotoxicity
5. Other:
    - Nausea and vomiting
    - Headache, dizziness
    - Excessive salivation
    - Iodism
    - Spastic contraction of the lower extremities.

REFERENCES

1. Allen, J. H., Parera, C., and Potts, D. G.: The relation of arterial trauma to complications of cerebral angiography. Amer. J. Roentgenol., 95:845-851, Dec. 1965.
2. Baum, S., Stein, G. N., and Kuroda, K. K.: Complications of "No Arteriography." Radiology, 86:835-838, May 1966.
3. Bartley, O., Bengtsson, U., and Cederbom, G.: Renal function before and after urography and angiography with large doses of contrast media. Acta Radiologica (Diag.), 8:9-16, Jan. 1969.
4. Bassett, F. H., Lincoln, C. R., King, T. D., and Canent, R. V.: Inequality in the size of the lower cardiac catheterizatio. Southern Med. J., 61:1013-1017, Oct. 1968.
5. Beall, A. C., Morris, G. C., Garrett, H. E., Henley, W. S., Hallman, G. L., Crawford, E. S., Cooley, D. A., and DeBakey, M. E.: Translumbar aortography; present indications and techniques. Ann. Int. Med., 60:843-856, May 1964.
6. Berdon, W. E., Schwartz, R. H., Becker, J., and Baker, D. H.: Tamm-Horsfall proteinuria. Radiology, 92:714-722, Mar. 1969.
7. Bernstein, E. F., Feinberg, S. B., and Greenspan, R. H.: Intravenous aortography. Surgery, 54:382-387, Aug. 1963.
8. Björk, L.: Effect of angiocardiography on erythrocyte aggregation in the conjunctival vessels. Acta Radiol. Diagn., 6:459-464, Sep. 1967.
9. Chase, N. E., and Kricheff, I. I.: The comparison of the complication rate of meglumine jothalamate and sodium diatrizoate in cerebral angiography. Amer. J. Roentgenol., 95:852-856, Dec. 1965.
10. Cohen, L. S., Kokko, J. P., and Williams, W. H.: Hemolysis and hemoglobinuria following angiography. Radiology, 92:329-332, Feb. 1969.
11. Cornell, S. H.: Spasticity of the lower extremities following abdominal aortography. Radiology, 93:377-379, Aug. 1969.
12. Doumanian, H. O., and Amplatz, K.: Vascular jet collapse in selective angiocardiography. Amer. J. Roentgenol., 100:344-352, June 1967.
13. Dudrick, S., Masland, W., and Mishkin, M.: Brachial plexus injury following axillary artery puncture. Radiology, 88:271-273, Feb. 1967.
14. Halpern, M.: Percutaneous transfemoral arteriography; an analysis of the complications in 1,000 consevutive cases. Amer. J. Roetgenol., 92:918-934, Oct. 1964.
15. Haut, G., and Amplatz, K.: Complication rates of transfemoral and transaortic catheterization. Surgery, 63:594-596, April 1968.
16. Hemley, S. D., Kanick, V., Kittredge, R. D., and Finby, N.: Intravenous aortography. Med. Radiogr. Photogr., 43:1-31, 1967.
17. Howland, W. J., Curry, J. L., and Wheeler, P. P.: Intra-arterial administration of procaine hydrochloride after arteriography; potential value in preventing arteriospasm and thrombosis. J.A.M.A., 201:813-816, Sept. 1967.
18. Jacobsson, B.: Effect of pretreatment with dextran 70 on platelet adhesiveness and thromboembolic complications following percutaneous arterial catherisation. Acta Radiological (Diag.), 8:289-295, July 1969.
19. Jacobsson, B., Paulin, S., and Schlossman, D.: Thromboembolism of leg following percutaneous

catheterisation of femoral artery for angiography. Acta Radiologica (Diag.), 8:97-108, March 1969.

20. Klatte, E. C., Brooks, A. L., and Rhamy, R. K.: Toxicity of intra-arterial barbiturates and tranquilizing drugs. Radiology, 92:700-704, Mar. 1969.
21. Killen, D. A., and Foster, J. H.: Spinal cord injury as a complication of contrast angiography. Surg., 59:969-981, June 1966.
22. Lang, E. K.: A survey of the complications of percutaneous retrograde arteriography; Seldinger technic. Radiology, 81:257-263, Aug. 1963.
23. Lang, E. K.: Prevention and treatment of complications following arteriography. Radiology, 88: 950-956, May, 1967.
24. Langsjoen, P. H., and Best, E. B.: Studies in the prevention of complications of angiography. Amer. J. Roetgenol., 106:425-433, June 1969.
25. Lasser, E. C.: *Dynamic Factors in Roentgen Diagnosis.* Baltimore, Williams & Wilkins, 1967.
26. Leadbetter, G. W., Jr., and Markland, C.: Evaluation of technics and complications of renal angiography. New Eng. J. Med., 266:10-13, Jan. 1962.
27. Lodin, H., and Ottander, H. G.: Technical puncture complications in carotid angiography. Brit. J. Radiology, 39:782-785, Oct. 1966.
28. McAfee, J. G.: A survey of complications of abdominal aortography. Radiology, 68:825-838, June 1957.
29. Mortensen, J. D.: Clinical sequelae from arterial needle puncture, cannulation and incision. Circulation, 35:1118-1123, June 1967.
30. Nebesar, R. A., and Pollard, J. J.: Catheter recoil and whipping in aortography. Radiology, 89:845-847, Nov. 1967.
31. Szilagyi, D. E., Smith, R. F., Macksood, A. J., and Eyler, W. R.: Abdominal aortography; its value and its hazards. Arch. Surg., 85:25-40, July 1962.
32. Taveras, J. M., and Wood, E. H.: *Diagnostic Neuroradiology.* Baltimore, Williams & Wilkins, 1964.

5

ANGIOGRAPHY OF TUMORS

THE DEGREE ANGIOGRAPHY CAN HELP with the diagnosis of a mass lesion varies with the lesion's vascular characteristics and its effect on surrounding vessels. Angiography is obviously more accurate with highly vascular tumors which present the eye with enlarged normal vessels, collateral vessels, neovasculature (irregularly branching and anastamosing vascular channels usually characterized by an appearance of tortuosity and/or irregular dilation and narrowing), and a rich, sharply or poorly marginated tissue "stain" in the arteriolar-capillary phase. Avascular lesions are more difficult to identify until they become gross, displacing normal vessels or structures, extending into the lumens of hollow organs, or being demonstrated as a "black" defect on the grey tissue background of the arteriolar-capillary phase of an angiographic study of a vascular organ. It is frustrating to realize some typically vascular tumors can be diffusely infiltrating or outgrow their blood supply, become necrotic and present as avascular lesions.

A table of the "typical" appearance of a group of lesions collected from the literature is appended. It is meant to suggest some possible indications and limitations of angiography and to aid in differential diagnosis.

For a time, it was hoped that the response of vessels to epinephrine might differentiate benign and maligant disease; however, there are both false negatives and false positives.

Very few neoplastic or inflammatory processes have vascular patterns which are truly unique. The appearance of primary renal carcinoma is typical in approximately two-thirds of cases (15) demonstrating increased local vascularity, hypertrophy of the feeding vessels, neovasculature and arterio-venous shunting. The angiographic appearance of metastatic renal carcinoma is usually identical to the primary lesion. Therefore, the finding of a renal lesion and multiple other visceral lesions of this description is almost pathognomonic of this condition; though it can be simulated by multiple primary lesions or conceivably multiple metastases to the kidney and other abdominal viscera (6).

Ilial carcinoid is one of the few tumors where the angiographic features alone have been proposed as pathognomonic. The angiographic complex put forward includes "a stellate arterial pattern, narrowing of deep mesenteric branches, poor-to-moderate accumulation of contrast medium, and non-visualization of veins" (13).

Most angiographic diagnoses of neoplasms are made by combining clinical, laboratory, and plain film information and the angiographic findings. In certain areas as the bladder and cervix, angiography is performed not to diagnose but to determine the gross extent or stage of the tumor.

Typically High Vascular

Hemangiomas, A.V. malformation
Pyogenic abscesses, acute and sub-acute
Active granulomatous disease
Carcinoid
Pheochromocytoma
Islet cell tumor
Meningioma
Renal angiofibrolipoma (tuberous sclerosis)
Glioblastoma multiforme
Melanoma
"Sarcomas"
Glomus tumors, angiofibromas
Hepatoma
Hypernephroma

Typically Avascular

Hematoma
Chronic and healed abscesses
"Healed" granulomas
Squamous cell carcinomas
Adrenal adenoma
Pancreatic carcinoma
Osteoma, fibromas, lipomas
Bowel and bladder polyps
Low grade gliomas, astrocytomas
Lymphoma
"Adenocarcinomas"
"Cysts"
Infarcts

Intermediate

Metastatic adenocarcinoma and squamous cell carcinoma
Transitional cell carcinoma
Wilm's

REFERENCES

1. Abrams, H. L.: The response of neoplastic renal vessels to epinephrine in man. Radiology, 82:217-224, Feb. 1964.
2. Abrams, R. M., Beranbaum, E. R., Beranbaum, S. L., and Ngo. N. L.: Angiographic studies of benign and malignant cystadenoma of the pancreas. Radiology, 89:1028-1032, Dec. 1967.
3. Abrams, R. M., Beranbaum, E. R., Santos, J. S., and Lipson, J.: Angiographic features of cavernous hemangioma of liver. Radiology, 92:308-313, Feb. 1969.
4. Boijsen, E., and Reuter, S. R.: Mesenteric angiography in the evaluation of inflammatory and neoplastic disease of the intestine. Radiology, 87:1028-1036, Dec. 1966.
5. Boijsen, E., Wallace, S., and Kanter, I. E.: Angiography in tumours of the stomach. Acta Radiologica (Diag.), 4:306-320, May 1966.
6. Bosniak, M. A., O'Connor, J. F., and Caplan, L. H.: Renal arteriography in patients with metastatic renal cell carcinoma. J.A.M.A., 203:249-254, Jan. 1968.
7. Clemett, A. R., and Park, W. M.: Arteriographic demonstration of pancreatic tumor in the Zollinger-Ellison syndrome. Radiology, 88:32-34, Jan. 1967.
8. Kahn, P. C., and Wise, H. M.: Simulation of renal tumor response to epinephrine by inflammatory disease. Radiology, 89:1062 1064, Dec. 1967.
9. Lagergren, C., and Lindbom, A.: Angiography of peripheral tumors. Radiology, 79:371-377, Sept. 1962.
10. McAlister, W. H., Margulis, A. R., Heinbecker, P., and Spjut, H.: Arteriography and microangiography of gastric and colonic lesions. Radiology, 79:769-782, Nov. 1962.
11. Nebesar, R. A., and Pollard, J. J.: A critical evaluation of selective celiac and superior mesenteric angiography in the diagnosis of pancreatic diseases, particularly malignant tumor; Facts and "artefacts," Radiology, 89:1017 1027, Dec. 1967.
12. Palmisano, P.: Renal hamartoma (angiomyolipoma). Radiology, 88:249-252, Feb. 1967.
13. Reuter, S. R., and Boijsen, E.: Angiographic findings in two ileal carcinoid tumors. Radiology, 87:836-840, Nov. 1969.
14. Reuter, S. R., Redman, H. C., and Siders, D. B.: The spectrum of angiographic findings in hepatoma. Radiology, 94:89-94, Jan. 1970.
15. Watson, R. C., Fleming, R. J., and Evans, J. A.: Arteriography in the diagnosis of renal carcinoma. Radiology, 91:888-897, Nov. 1968.

6

ANGIOGRAPHY OF ISCHEMIA

THE QUANTITATIVE DETERMINATION OF BLOOD FLOW by angiography is a long sought dream that has yet to enter the clinical realm, although some inroads are made by each generation of physicians and equipment.

One basic problem underlying the present day problem is the pharmacologic effect of modern media on blood flow. No matter how sophisticated the equipment and technique, media induced vasomotor activity removes the result from the "physiologic realm." Mechanically induced vasospasm will also haunt the data so long as it is necessary to place a needle or catheter selectively into the vessel under study to obtain the best contrast and delineation of vascular anatomy. Despite these nuances, practical information is obtainable.

Occlusions. Acute, uncompensated complete obstruction is evidenced by a cut-off, an arrest of an opacified column of blood proximal to the site of obstruction, with poor or no significant collateral vessels and no visualization downstream. The cut-off is recognized by filling of branches of parallel, similar sized or smaller vessels beyond the channel in question as well as a temporal delay. This sign is based on the observations that the appearance time (apparent speed of flow) is always more rapid in larger channels than smaller channels. Marked vasospasm, compression of arteries by increased pressure of surrounding tissues, occluding embolus as well as thrombosis, can present with the same picture. In end arteries, the localization of the site of obstruction can be falsely portrayed by an arrest of the column of contrast proximally where active flow ceases (2, 6).

Acute obstruction of a chronically stenosed vessel and chronic localized obstruction present a similar picture with: (1) a cut-off, and (2) existing collaterals shunting blood around the obstructed site and re-opacifying the vessel distally.

An auxiliary sign of acute or chronic obstruction which is useful in some areas is the lack of normal tissue straining in the "capillary phase" of highly vascular organs (as kidney, myocardium, spleen, etc.). In organs of intermediate vascularity as brain, subtraction of properly timed, high quality radiographs can demonstrate large avascular areas of parenchyma.

Stenoses. Predicting significance of stenoses is more difficult than diagnosing occlusion. The basis of interpretation goes back to a number of biophysical experiments thirty years ago which demonstrated the degree to which an elastic vessel has to be compromised to create a pressure gradient and diminish flow. The factors influencing this phenomena are the length and other physical characteristics of the lesion, the viscosity of the blood as well as the degree of encroachment on the lumen. The anatomic severity of stenoses are usually estimated by the estimation of the mean minimum diameter (preferably averaged in two planes) as compared to the mean diameter above and below the lesion. In case of a lesion at a vessel origin, this calculation is made by comparing the minimum diameter of the lesion versus the diameter of the vessel distally (prior to branching) or versus the diameter of the opposite corresponding artery where there is a reasonable probability of original symmetry.

Presuming a cylindrical stenosis (the length of which approximates the lumen diameter) in a cylindrical elastic tube, the minimum encroachment on the lumen which would affect flow is a reduction of approximately 50 per cent in diameter (75 per cent in lumen area). To accomplish a 50 per cent reduction in flow, a reduction of about 70 per cent in diameter (or 90 per cent in lumen area) is necessary.

Other signs which are useful in evaluating stenoses are: (1) the presence of collaterals; (2) the rapidity of flow in the vessel under consideration versus parallel, similar or smaller sized vessels; (3) post-stenotic dilatation; (4) prolongation of opacification of the vessel distal to the stenosis due to sluggish flow. The internal cerebral circulation, the circulation of the stomach, the gut, the pelvic organs and the pancreas usually possess functional rather than potential anastamosis of medium sized arteries. Therefore, a changing pattern of flow can be seen physiologically in these vessels; (5) a reversal in the direction of flow in an end artery can be evidence of a severe stenosis or occlusion ("steal syndrome"), and (6) the size and function of an organ can reflect the importance of a stenotic lesion, particularly if the size can be documented as previously normal and there has been no intervening inflammatory or degenerative process. In the kidney, the renal vein pressor substances can be assayed. In the heart (or any organ), the lactate and pyruvate in the venous return can give an estimate of oxidative metabolism (7). A pressure gradient across a stenosis is a classical and accurate method of estimating severity and should be used more by arteriographers. However, the catheter's external diameter versus the size of the vessel lumen must be considered if the downstream pressure is measured with the catheter through the stenosis.

Artefacts. The negative side pressure sucking in the walls of a vessel adjacent to a high speed jet can produce the appearance of a stenosis (1). This is readily produced by a medium sized end-opening catheter in a medium sized artery during a high-speed injection. It can be seen with end and side hole catheters, but not with side holes only. Standing waves which produce a temporary symmetrically corrugated appearance also occur and such an appearance also calls for a repeat study.

Spasm can be induced by mechanical irritation of an arterial wall by any type of catheter. Any smooth stenosis of a medium sized artery where a catheter is or has just been, is suspect and should be verified with a second look (3, 5).

Unexplained areas of spasm can and do occur in the cerebral vessels, the coronaries, and probably other arteries. Some angiographers routinely employ nitroglycerine prior to coronary arteriography. Spasmolytics in other vessels are currently out of fashion, probably due to the low recognized frequency of this problem.

REFERENCES

1. Doumanian, H. O., and Amplatz, K.: Vascular jet collapse in selective angiocardiography. Amer. J. Roentgenol., 100:344-352, June 1967.
2. Ivan, L. P., and Marian, J. J.: Angiographic occlusive patterns of the internal carotid artery. J. Neurosurg., 30:233-237. Mar. 1969.
3. Lehrer, H.: The physiology of angiographic arterial waves. Radiology, 89:11-19, July 1967.
4. Mann, F. C.: Effect on blood flow of decreasing the lumen of blood vessel. Surgery 4:249-252, Aug. 1938.
5. New, P. F. J.: Arterial stationary waves. Amer. J. Roentgenol., 97:488-499, June 1966.
6. Newton, T. H., and Couch, R. S. C.: Possible errors in the arteriographic diagnosis of internal carotid artery occlusion. Radiology, 75:766-773, Nov. 1960.
7. Olin, T., and Redman, H.: Spillover flowmeter a preliminary report. Acta Radiologica (Diag.), 4:217-222, Mar. 1966.

7

TECHNIQUE OUTLINES

A. PRE-STUDY ORDERS

1. The primary operator is responsible for obtaining "informed consent" (1). In elective cases this means seeing the patient the day before or certainly before any sedation is administered.
2. Where sedation is indicated, the sedative can usually be given *orally* 1½ to 2 hours prior to the procedure. Intramuscularly, injections should be given 45 minutes prior to the procedure. In the average adult patient with normal liver and renal function premedication consists of: diazepam (Valium®) 5 to 10 mg or secobarbital (Seconal®) 100 mg — orally or intramuscularly;
   Atropine 0.4 — 0.6 mg
   ± meperidine (Demerol®) 50-100 mg } intramuscularly
3. A liquid or low residue diet for one or more days prior to examination and a cathartic the day before the procedure is important to abdominal angiography.
4. Dehydration is *contraindicated* preparatory to all angiography. A liquid diet can be employed up to 4 hours prior to the procedure (with normal gastric emptying). Intravenous fluids are indicated in dehydrated patients *prior* to media injection. Low molecular weight dextran should be considered in high risk patients.
5. Appropriate skin prep.

B. THE SELDINGER TECHNIQUE

Setting Up

1. Most patients undergoing angiography should be monitored by EKG. All high risk patients and any patient under-going catheterization of the ascending aorta should be monitored.
2. Wash powder off gloves in glove basin before setting up.
3. Check length of guide wire and catheter before beginning, to be sure wire is longer. Also check needle to be sure wire will go through, butt first.
4. Add 2 cc of Heparin 1:1000 to approximately 250 cc of normal saline or 5% glucose (cardiac) for flush solution.
5. To prevent fiber embolism, cotton sponges are not placed in "flush" basin. Use separate wash basin or preferably a "closed system."
6. Flush catheter and needle with heparin solution before inserting.

The Arterial Puncture

1. Do femoral arterial puncture at or just below the inguinal ligament. Near vertically oriented routes of puncture, particularly far below the inguinal ligament, cause difficult catheter control and frequently significant arterial damage.
2. In the emaciated patient, the needle is best stuck almost parallel to the femoral artery. With more fat the angle will approximate 45°.
3. In extreme obesity the artery is only palpable (and stickable) at the inguinal ligament. Don't go above it. Hemorrhages above this area go intraperitoneal, therefore are hard to detect early and hard to control.
4. Do not use so much local anesthetic that the artery is completely obscured to palpation. Excess anesthetic (as well as hematoma) can be kneaded away. The pain fibers in the arterial wall can't always be anesthetized, so there will usually be some pain on arterial puncture.
5. Nick the skin (2 mm cut) with an #11 scalpel blade. Spread with hemostat and see fat to be sure the incision is through all skin layers (plastic catheters drag on skin otherwise).
6. If you can't get a good pulsatile arterial flow after a stick, check with test dose of contrast medium and TV to see needle's relationship to vessel.

The Wire

1. Use teflon J wires for tortuous vessels and discard after procedure (2, 3, 4). Kifa wire may be used for good arteries and saved unless damaged. Check wire for kinks and roughness at tip. Check wire, catheter and needle for fit.
2. Fluoroscope the wire if it doesn't go immediately and easily. Don't jam wire. Start over if it won't go easily.
3. If possible, pass guide wire to distal aorta before introducing catheter.

The Catheter

1. With other than teflon catheters, dilate vessel puncture with a teflon dilator before attempting to put the catheter over the guide wire. (This maneuver may increase bleeding but doesn't require excessive pressure which can kink wire as catheter is inserted.)
2. Pass the catheter over the guide wire with short close strokes to prevent buckling of wire.
3. Aspirate when guide wire is removed to make certain of free flow of blood. Flush with heparinized saline and do not aspirate again except for sampling.
4. Keep catheters filled with contrast media or drip continuously to prevent clots.

The Injection

1. *Always* test proposed injection sites with 60% meglumine medium (by hand) with visualization before definitive dose. Alter dose and rate of contrast injection and rate and length of filming according to observed run-off.
2. Check injector syringe for air bubbles, media type, injector program and safety stop.

3. Usual maximum dose is 1 cc/lb Renografin 76% in adults with normal renal function (1.25 cc/lb Renografin 60%).
4. *Remember:* end-opening catheters (no side holes) recoil with jet phenomena.
   End and side-opening whip (particularly near their maximum injection rates).
   Side openings alone are most stable (can be introduced via sheath). Any dose rate can recoil a selectively placed catheter if the dose rate of dye greatly exceed the blood flow rate. (Look at the TV and go slow with stenosis, fast with rapid run-off).

Complications During the Procedures

1. Judgment must be exercised as to the number of sticks an artery can tolerate, and as to whether to continue with the same vessel after a wire or catheter is passed extraluminally
2. Syncopal or near syncopal episodes should be treated promptly by lowering the patient's head, raising his feet, and having the patient sniff strong aromatic ammonia.
3. Cardiac arrest must be treated immediately with proper resuscitation. For success, the emergency assignments of the special procedure personnel should be made and roles rehearsed.

C. TRANSLUMBAR CATHETERIZATION OF THE ABDOMINAL AORTA

1. Localize a point 1 to 2 cm below the left 12th rib, 10 to 12 cm lateral to the midline with film or fluoroscopic technique.
2. Make a 3 mm incision and probe with a curved hemostat to see fat.
3. Introduce an appropriately long sheath needle aiming obliquely toward the centrum of T 12.
4. When the needle touches bone, verify its position with film or fluoroscopy —then withdraw 5 cm and re-direct more vertically to miss the vertebral body.
5. Insert slowly, feeling for the aortic pulsation on the needle hub. Penetrate the aortic wall with a short controlled stab (1 cm thrust). A definite sensation of the puncture is usually felt.
6. Remove the stylet. If a pulsatile blood flow is not apparent, slowly withdraw (the needle tip may impinge on the far wall).
7. When a satisfactory flow is present, withdraw the needle and test with a small manually injected bolus of medium and either fluoroscopy or a film as a check of position of the sheath.
8. The sheath's position can be manipulated with curved guide wire, or guide wire tip deflector device.

D. BRACHIAL CUT-DOWN

1. Make the incision transversely at least 4 cm in length or wider in obese arms.
2. Take care to use adequate local anesthetic to prevent arterial spasm.
3. After the vessel is exposed, run gently under it with a curved hemostat to check for posterior branches.

4. Place tapes soaked in anesthetic, or rubber bands above and below the site of arteriotomy and clean the adventia from the site to be opened (to make repair easier).
5. Keep tapes (if used) and wound moist by irrigating the wound intermittenly (with anesthetic if spasm is problem).
6. Inject 500 units of heparin in 5 cc of saline into vessel and tighten tapes to occlude flow.
7. Make arterial opening with opthalmolgic scissors or a fine blade, and probe wound with fine opthalmologic pick-ups or special rake. Insert catheter into true lumen through jaws of pick-ups or with rake releasing proximal tape or band. Re-tighten and clamp tapes snugly.
8. Remove the catheter after the procedure and check for back bleeding by momentarily releasing distal tape. If back bleeding absent or diminished, use Fogerty catheter or similar device to remove distal clot.
9. It is usually necessary to repair the artery following cut-down since adequate hemostasis is difficult to obtain following interruption of the subcutaneous tissues.

E. POST-PROCEDURE CARE

1. After removing the needle or catheter, hold gentle, firm, *continuous* pressure over the site of arterial repair or puncture for 5 to 10 minutes. Observe the distal extremity for color and pulse. Don't obliterate pulse with too much pressure. Unless carefully used, C-clamps can increase the rate of thrombosis.
2. The alert, reasonable patient is his own best nurse in the immediate post-angiographic period, and should be *informed* how to temporarily treat delayed hemorrhage, hematoma formation from the needle or catheter entry site. Talk to him.
3. Patients who have any complication, and patients in whom a complication is expected must be sent to a recovery room. It is desirable for all patients to be in a recovery room for 2 to 4 hours after the procedure. A sandbag over a femoral artery wound may be helpful to keep patients still, as well as to continue pressure.
4. Post-operative care should include:
   a. Resume former medications and diet. Force fluids.
   b. Bed rest for 12 to 24 hours.
   c. Checking of wounds for bleeding or swelling, and pulses, color and temperature of the extremity distal to the site of puncture (punctures). In the usual case, the extremity and the patient's blood pressure should be checked every 30 minutes for 4 to 6 hours.
   d. In case of bleeding or increasing hematoma formation, hold gentle but firm manual pressure over site and contact radiologist.
   e. Immediately contact radiologist for pallor, pulselessness, or pain in the extremity distal to the site of puncture.
   f. Remove any bandage employed the following morning.

REFERENCES

1. Collins, V. P.: Consent to radiologic examinations. Radiology, 91:85-91, July, 1968.
2. Judkins, M. P., Hinck, V. C., and Dotter, C. T.: Teflon-coated safety guides; an adjunct to the

use of polyurethane catheters. Amer. J. Roentgenol., 104:223-224, Sept. 1968.

3. Judkins, M. P., Kidd, H. J., Frische, L. H., and Dotter, C. T.: Lumen-following safety J-guide for catheterization of tortuous vessels. Radiology, 88:1127-1130, June 1967.
4. Nebesar, R. A., and Pollard, J. J.: A curved tip guide wire for thoracic and abdominal angiography. Amer. J. Roentgenol., 97:508-510, June 1966.
5. Standen, J. R., Nogrady, M. B., Dunbar, J. S., and Goldbloom, R. B.: The osmotic effects of methylglucamine diatrizoate (Renografin 60) in intravenous urography in infants. Amer. J. Roengenol., 93:473-479, Feb. 1965.

CENTRAL NERVOUS SYSTEM

Carotid Arteriorgram

TRAY — Angiogram and 12″ PE 320 polyethylene (soft) connector, or Seldinger tray.

NEEDLE — 18 gauge arteriographic or sheath, or "headhunter" catheter (Judkins design).

OPAQUE MEDIA — 60% meglumine diatrizoate or iothalamate.

INJECTION RATE — 4-6 cc/sec for 1.5 to 2 sec.

FILM RATE — 1. Routine — 2/sec for 2 sec then 1/sec for 5 sec.
2. Rapid flow sequence (for A-V malformation, abnormal isotope flow study, and intracranial occlusion disease) — 3/sec for 3 sec then 1/sec for 4 sec.
3. Cerebral aneurysm localization (oblique position) — 2/sec for 2 sec. (Start changer at beginning of injection).

NOTES

If a shift of midline structures is present and a subdural is suspected, do obliques in addition to routine "AP" and lateral as subdural collections far anterior or posterior are sometimes difficult to see. Choose appropriate oblique by the position of the anterior cerebral artery and internal cerebral vein. If there is more posterior shift, turn the face away from the enlarged hemisphere.

Percutaneous puncture of the carotid is performed as for other vessels except that local anesthetic can be infiltrated posterior to the carotid to raise the vessel and help to fix it. The common carotid is punctured about two finger breadths above the medial border of the clavicle. Internal carotid puncture is more cephalad and is attempted where the best pulsation is palpated in the neck. When the vessel is punctured, the needle is threaded into the artery with a guide wire or protruding blunt obturator. The obturator is replaced with a syringe and connectors filled with meglumine diatrizoate or iothalamate 60% for a small test injection by hand to be checked by TV or Polaroid film. After the injection, the blunt obturator is replaced while the films are checked. The adult circulation time (time difference between the points of maximum concentration in the carotid siphon and in the parietal veins) is 4.13 sec according to Greitz (2).

REFERENCES

1. DiChiro, G.: Angiographic patterns of cerebral convexity veins and superficial dural sinuses. Amer. J. Roentgenol., 87:308-321, Feb. 1962.
2. Greitz, T.: A radiologic study of the brain circulation by rapid serial angiography of the carotid artery. Acta Radiologica: Suppl., 140, 1956.
3. Hinck, V. C., Judkins, M. P., and Paxton, H. D.: Simplified selective femorocerebral angiography. Radiology, 89:1048-1052, Dec. 1967.
4. Jimenez, J. P., and Goree, J. A.: The normal middle cerebral artery axis. Amer. J. Roentgenol., 101:88-93, Sept. 1967.
5. Lodin, H., and Ottander, H. G.: Technical puncture complications in carotid angiography. Brit. J.. Radiol., 39:782-785, Oct. 1966.
6. Meschan, I.: Roentgen Signs of Abnormality in Cerebral Angiograms. In: *Special Techiques for Neurological Diagnosis,* edited by James F. Toole, Philadelphia, Davis, 1969, ch. 6, pp. 94-137.
7. Taveras, J. M., and Wood, E. H.: *Diagnostic Neuroradiology.* Baltimore,, Williams & Wilkins, 1964.

8. Wallace, S., Goldberg, H. I., Leeds, N. E., and Mishkin, M. M.: The cavernous branches of the internal carotid artery. Amer J. Roentgenol., 101:34-46, Sept. 1967.
9. Wilson, M.: *Anatomical Foundation of Neuroradiology of the Brain.* Boston, Little, Brown, 1963.
10. Wollschlaeger, G., Wollschlaeger, P. B., Lucus, F., and Lopez, V. F.: Experience and result with postmortem cerebral angiography performed as routine procedure of the autopsy. Amer. J. Roentgenol., 101:68-87, Sept. 1967.

NOTES

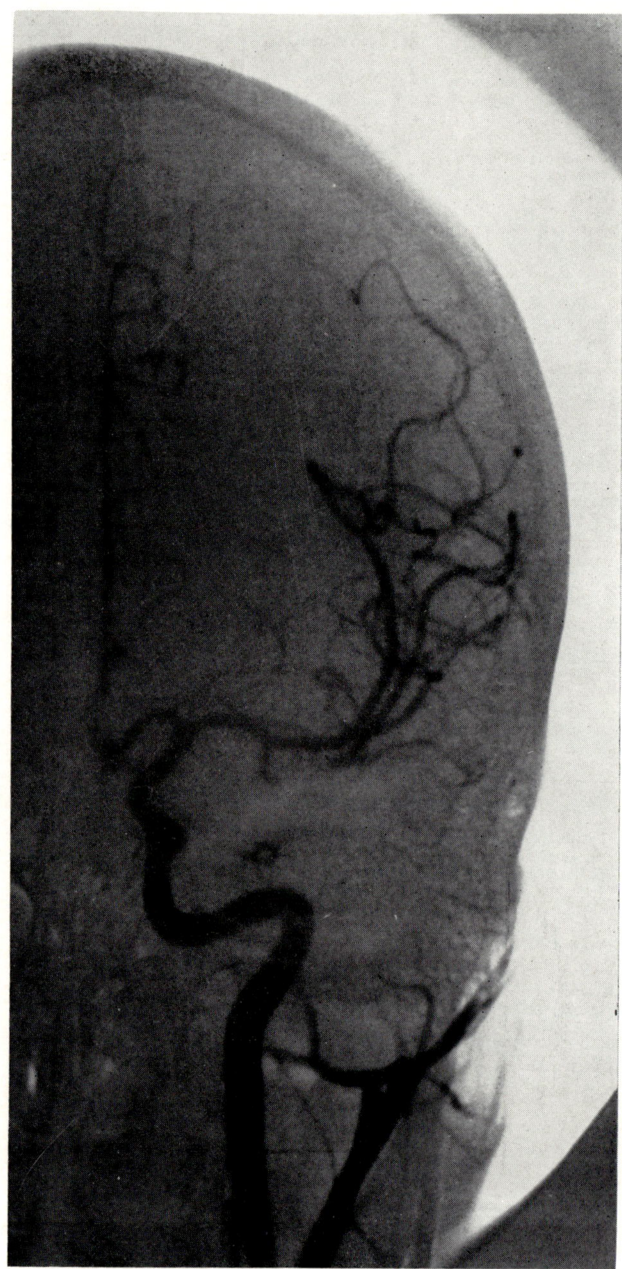

FIGURE 1. Carotid Arteriogram (Anterior-posterior projection).

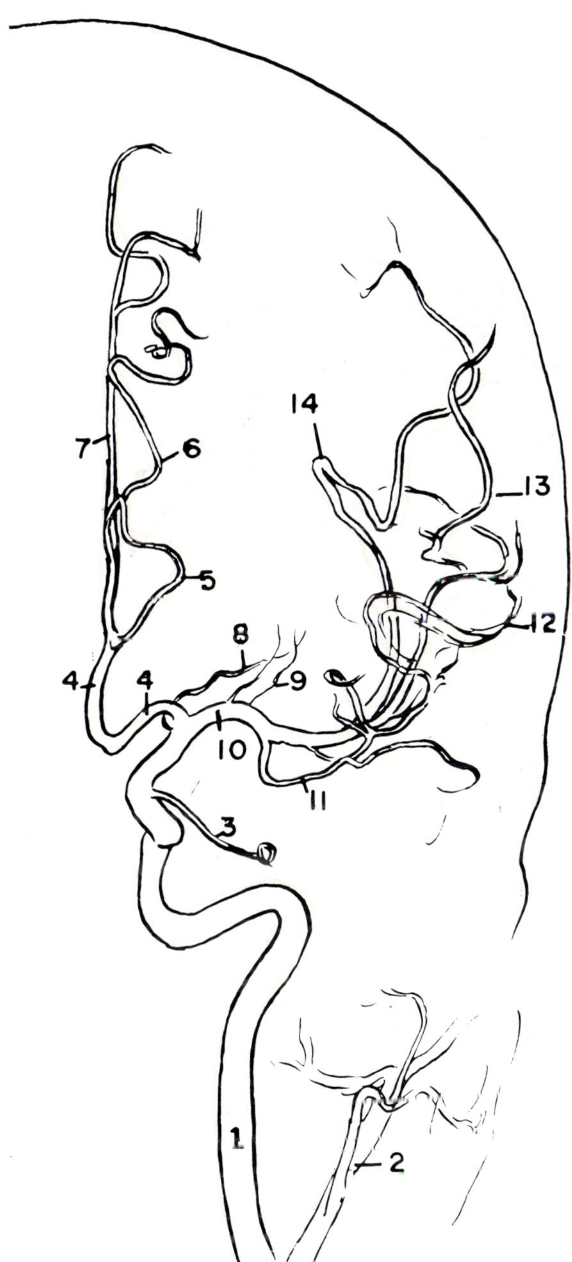

1. Internal carotid A.
2. External carotid A.
3. Ophthalmic A.
4. Anterior cerebral A.
5. Frontopolar A.
6. Callosomarginal A.
7. Pericallosal A.
8. Anterior choroidal A.
9. Lenticulostriate A.
10. Middle cerebral A.
11. Ascending frontoparietal A.
12. Posterior temporal A. from middle cerebral A.
13. Angular A.
14. Posterior parietal A.

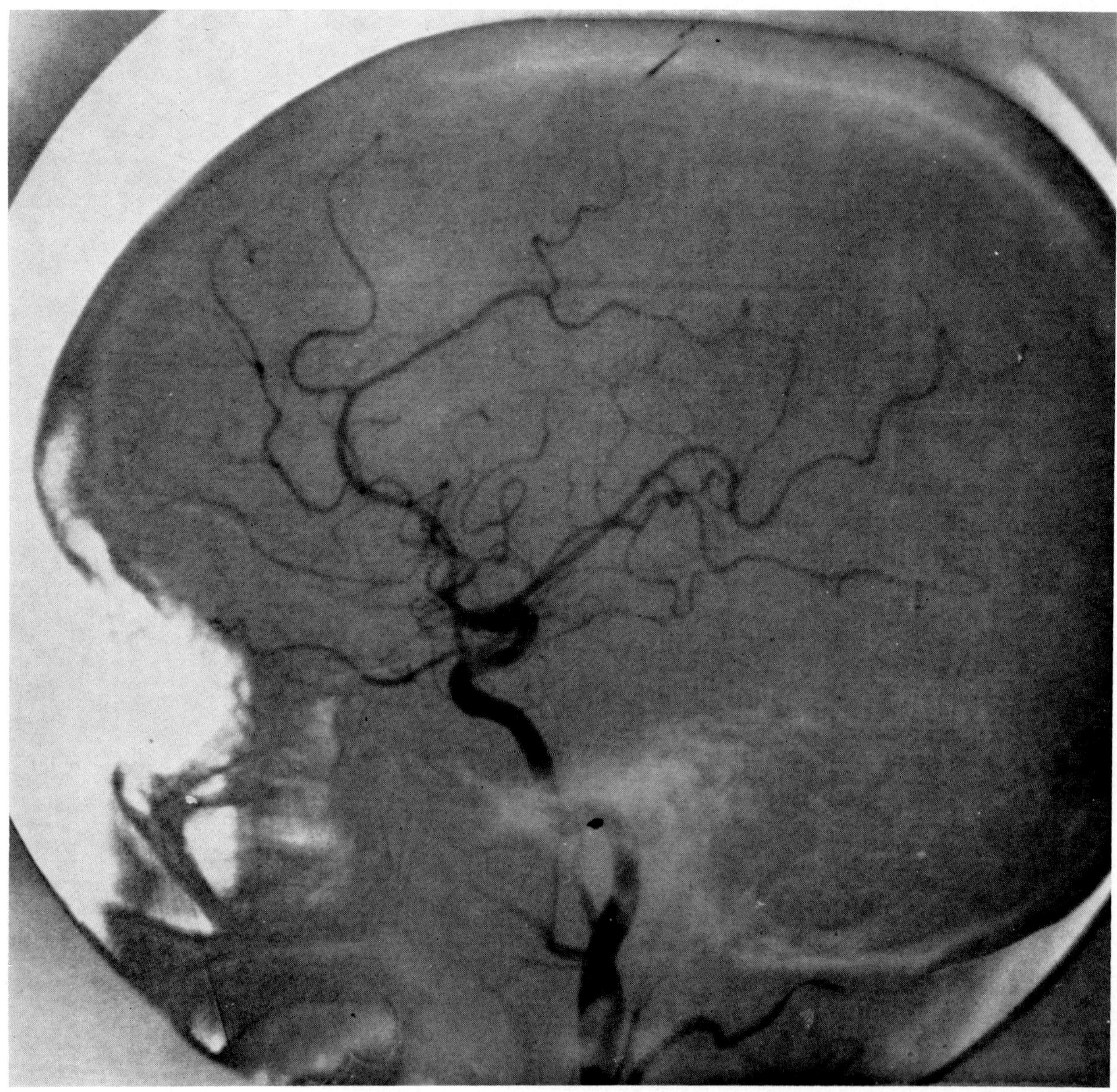

FIGURE 2. Carotid Arteriogram (Lateral projection).

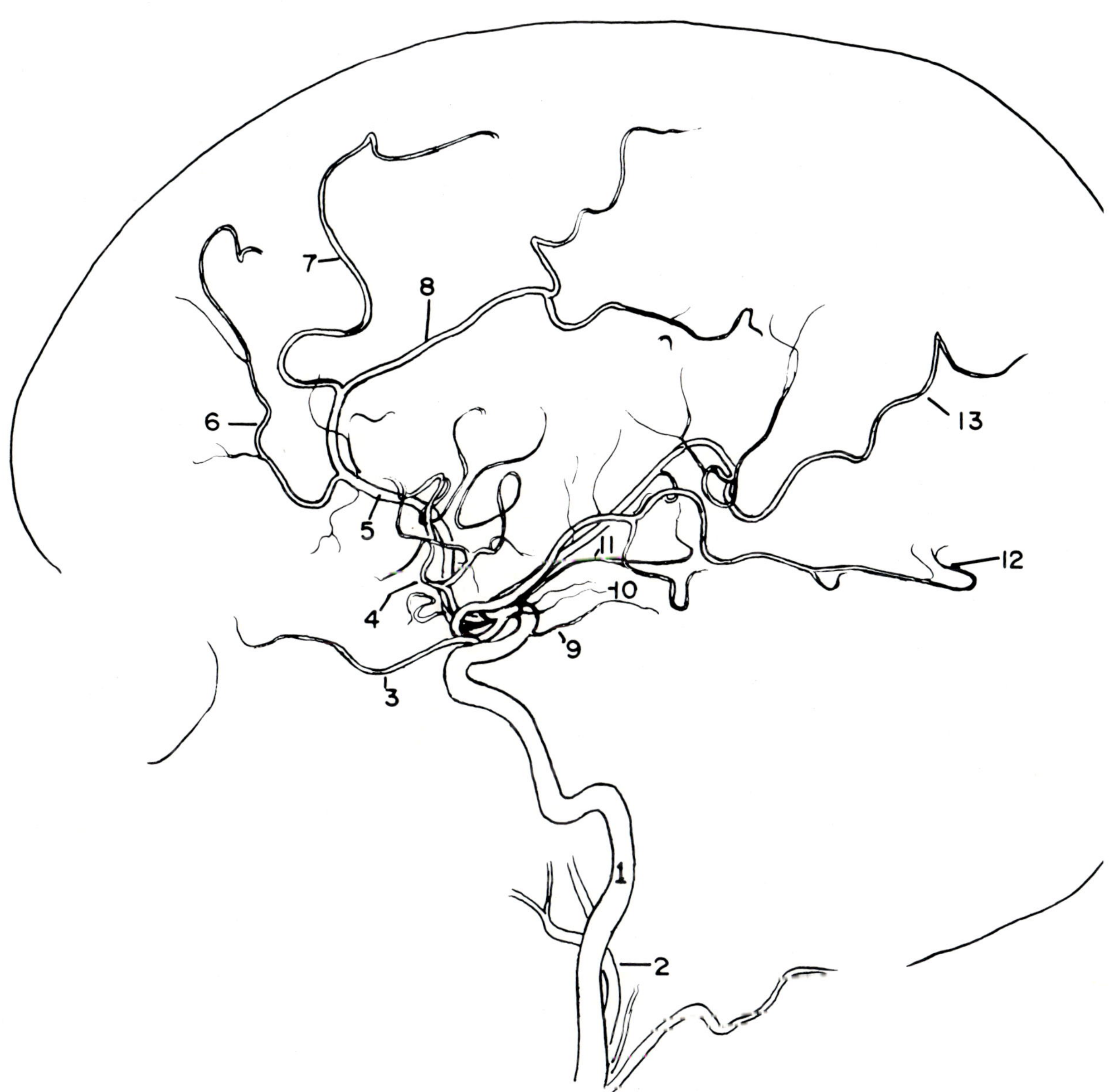

1. Internal carotid A.
2. External carotid and branches
3. Ophthalmic A.
4. Ascending frontoparietal A.
5. Anterior cerebral A.
6. Frontopolar A.
7. Callosomarginal
8. Pericallosal A.
9. Anterior choroidal A.
10. Lenticulostriate A.
11. Posterior temporal A. from middle cerebral A.
12. Angular A.
13. Posterior parietal A.

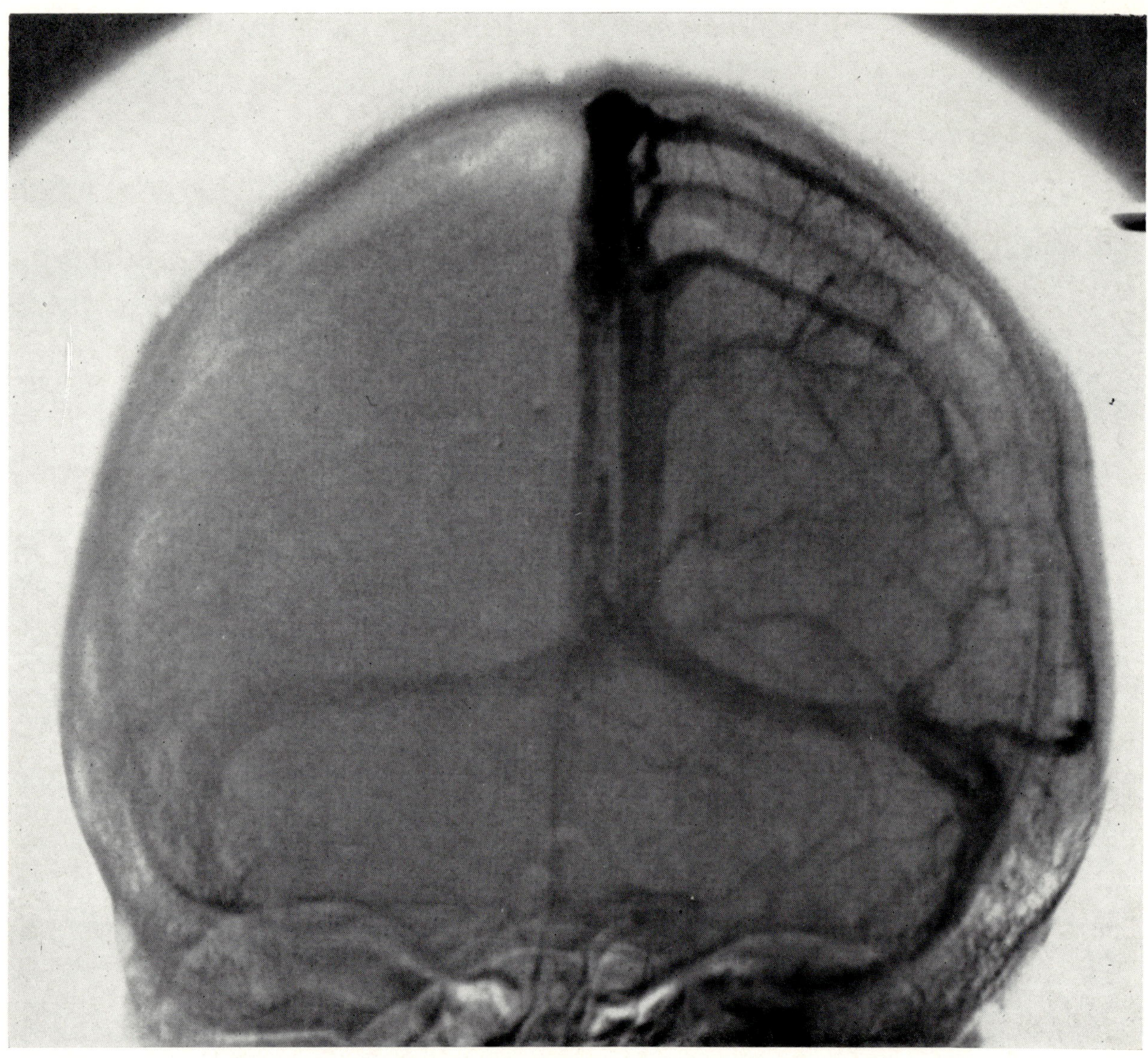

FIGURE 3. Cerebral Venogram (Anterior-posterior projection).

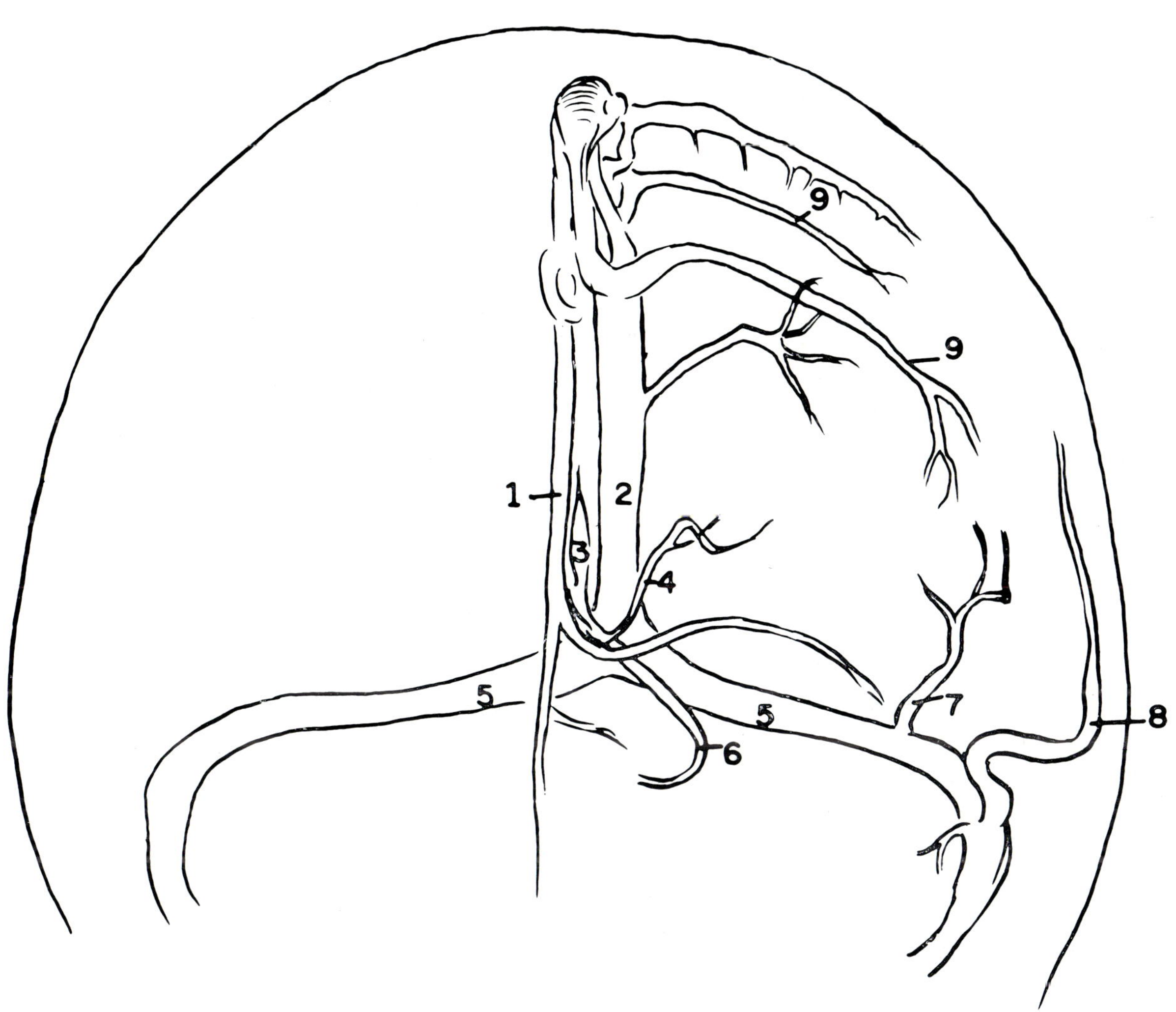

1. Superior sagittal sinus (anteriorly)
2. Superior sagittal sinus (posteriorly)
3. Internal cerebral vein
4. Striothalamic vein
5. Transverse sinus
6. Basal vein of Rosenthal
7. Inferior anastomotic vein of Labbé
8. Superficial middle cerebral vein
9. Superficial vein

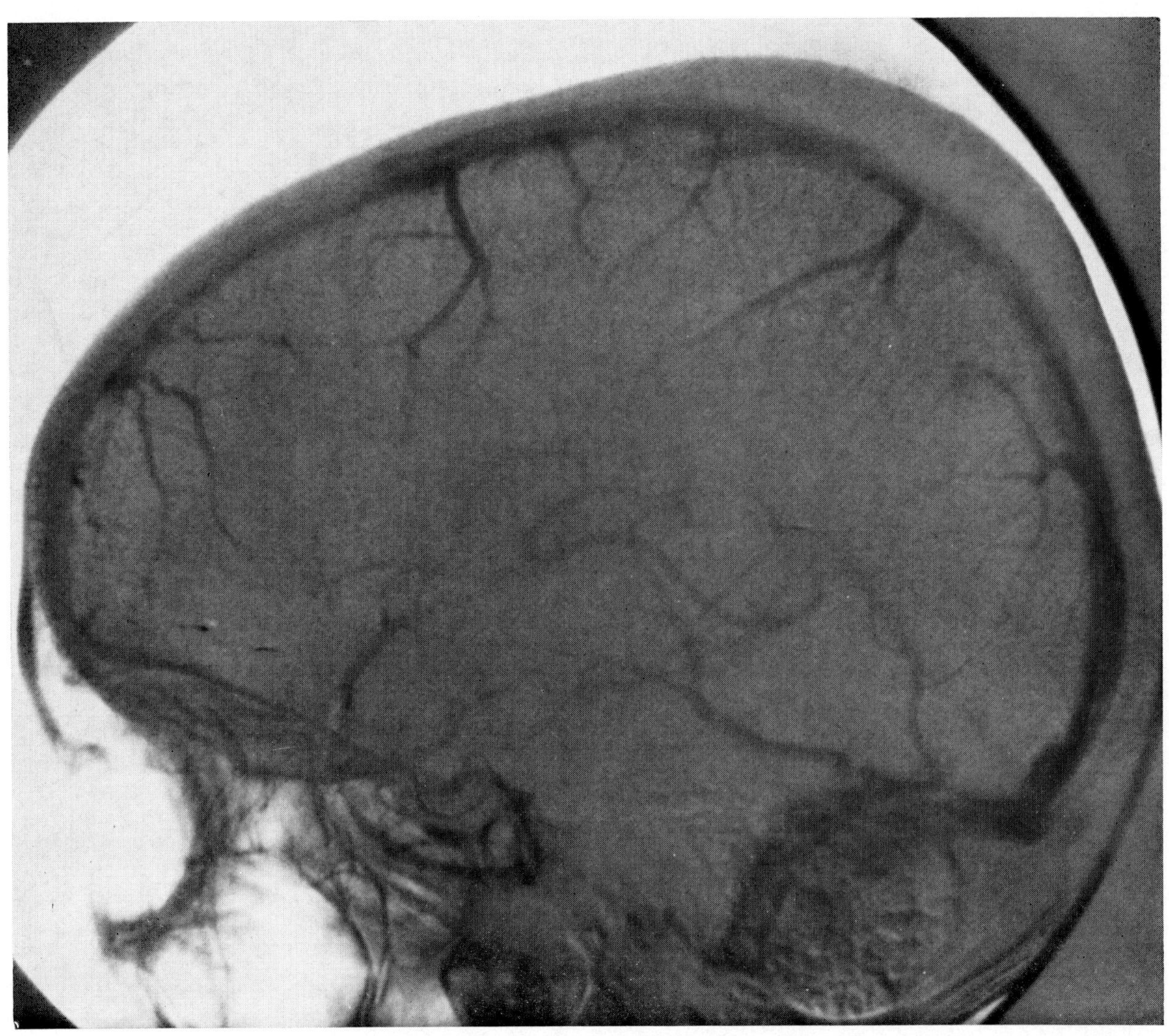

FIGURE 4. Cerebral Venogram (Lateral projection).

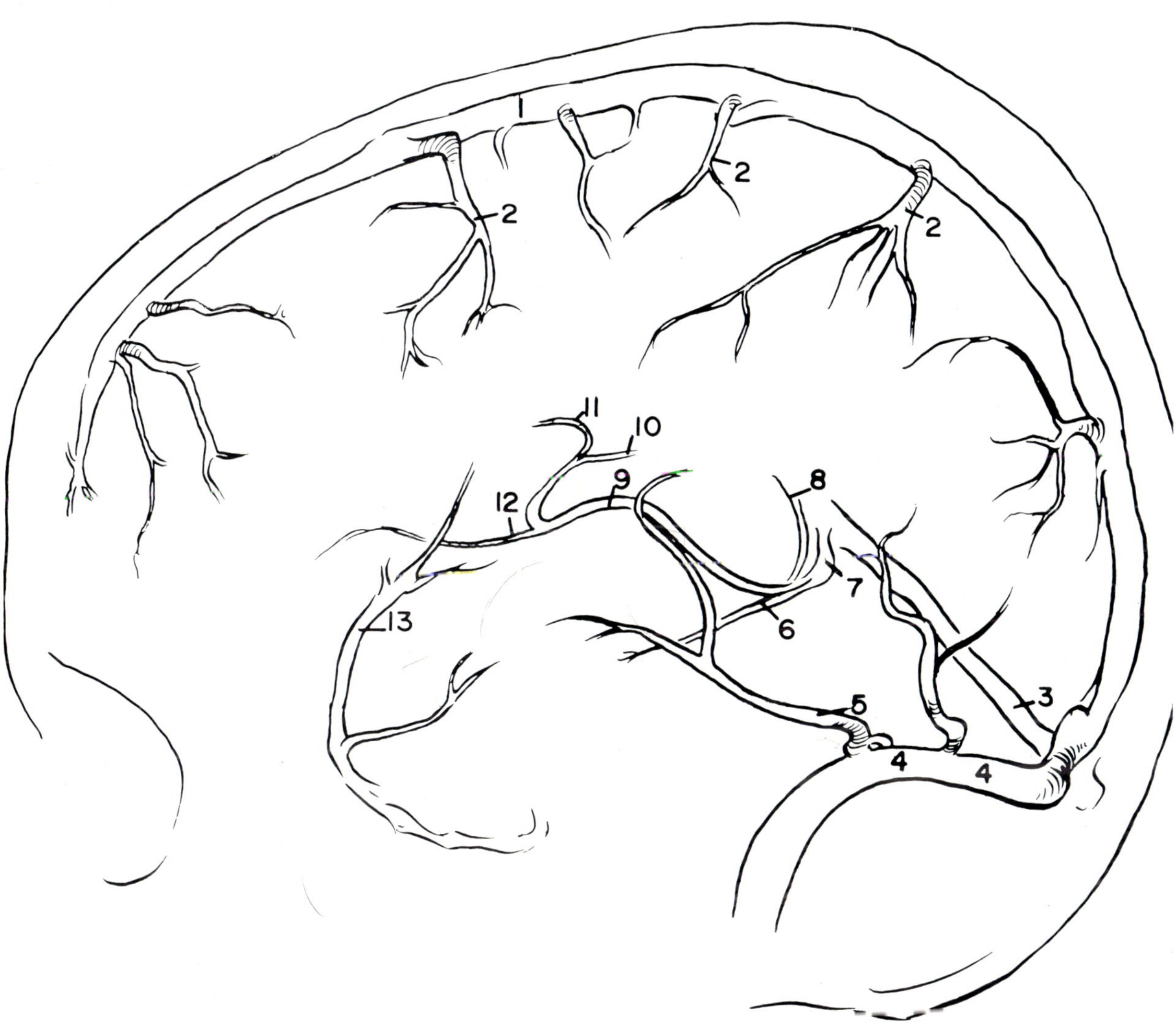

1. Superior sagittal sinus
2. Superficial vein
3. Straight sinus
4. Transverse sinus
5. Inferior anastomotic vein of Labbé
6. Basal vein of Rosenthal
7. Great cerebral vein of Galen
8. Posterior pericallosal vein
9. Internal cerebral vein
10. Striothalamic vein
11. Caudate vein
12. Septal vein
13. Superficial middle cerebral vein

External Carotid Arteriogram

TRAY — Angiogram
NEEDLE — Angiographic needle and short #4 catheter or sheath needle.
GUIDEWIRE — Precurved (short 0.035 in diameter)
OPAQUE MEDIA — 60% meglumine diatrizoate or iothalamate
INJECTION RATE — 2-4 cc/sec for 1.5 to 2 sec.
FILM RATE — 1/sec for 7 sec (A-V malformations 2/sec for 3 sec, then 1/sec for 4 sec).

NOTES

The common carotid is punctured low in the neck after infiltration with a local anesthetic. A test injection of 2 to 4 cc of contrast media is done and a lateral film of the neck made during injection, or horizontal beam lateral fluoroscopy is done. The exact location of the carotid bifurcation is visualized on this film. If there are no interfering stenotic lesions or atheromatous plaques, a guidewire is introduced through the needle followed by removal of the needle and introduction of the catheter or the sheath is advanced from sheath needle. The external carotid is anterior and medial to the internal carotid and with the curved guidewire the catheter tip can usually be directed into either the internal or the external carotid.

REFERENCES

1. Newton, T. H., and Kramer, R. A.: Clinical uses of selective external carotid arteriography. Amer. J. Roentgenol., 97:458-472, June 1966.
2. Pribram, H. F. W.: Selective catheterization of the external carotid artery. Radiology, 87:315-320, Aug. 1966.
3. Schechter, M. M.: Percutaneous carotid catheterization. Acta Radiologica (Diag.), 1:417-426, 1963.
4. Weidner, W., and Hanafee, W.: Selective external carotid angiography. Acta Radiologica (Diag.), 4:177-186, Mar. 1966.
5. Wilson, G., Weidner, W., and Hanafee, W.: The demonstration and diagnosis of meningiomas by selective carotid angiography. Amer. J. Roentgenol., 95:868-873, Dec. 1965.

NOTES

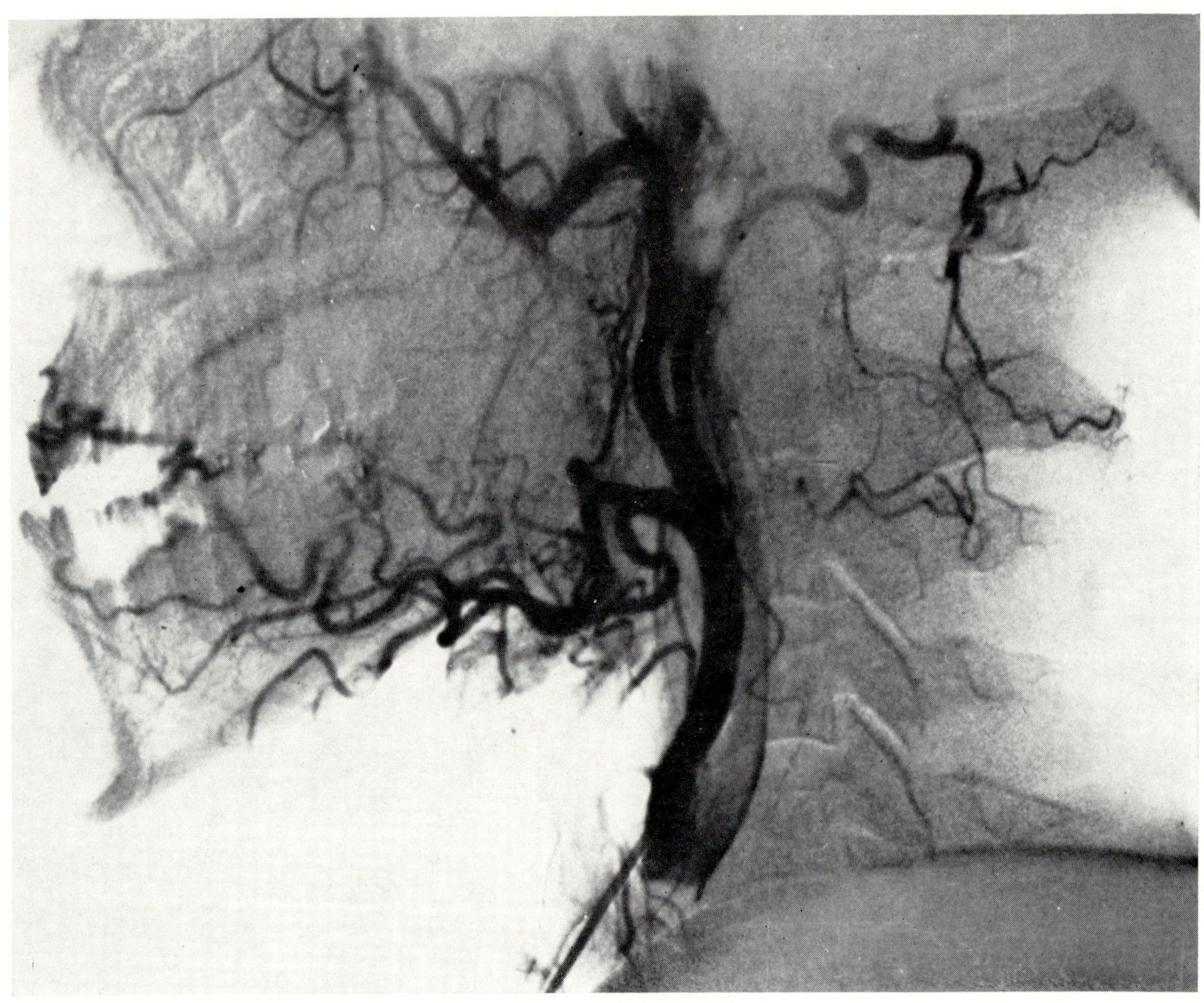

FIGURE 5. External Carotid Arteriogram (Lateral projection).

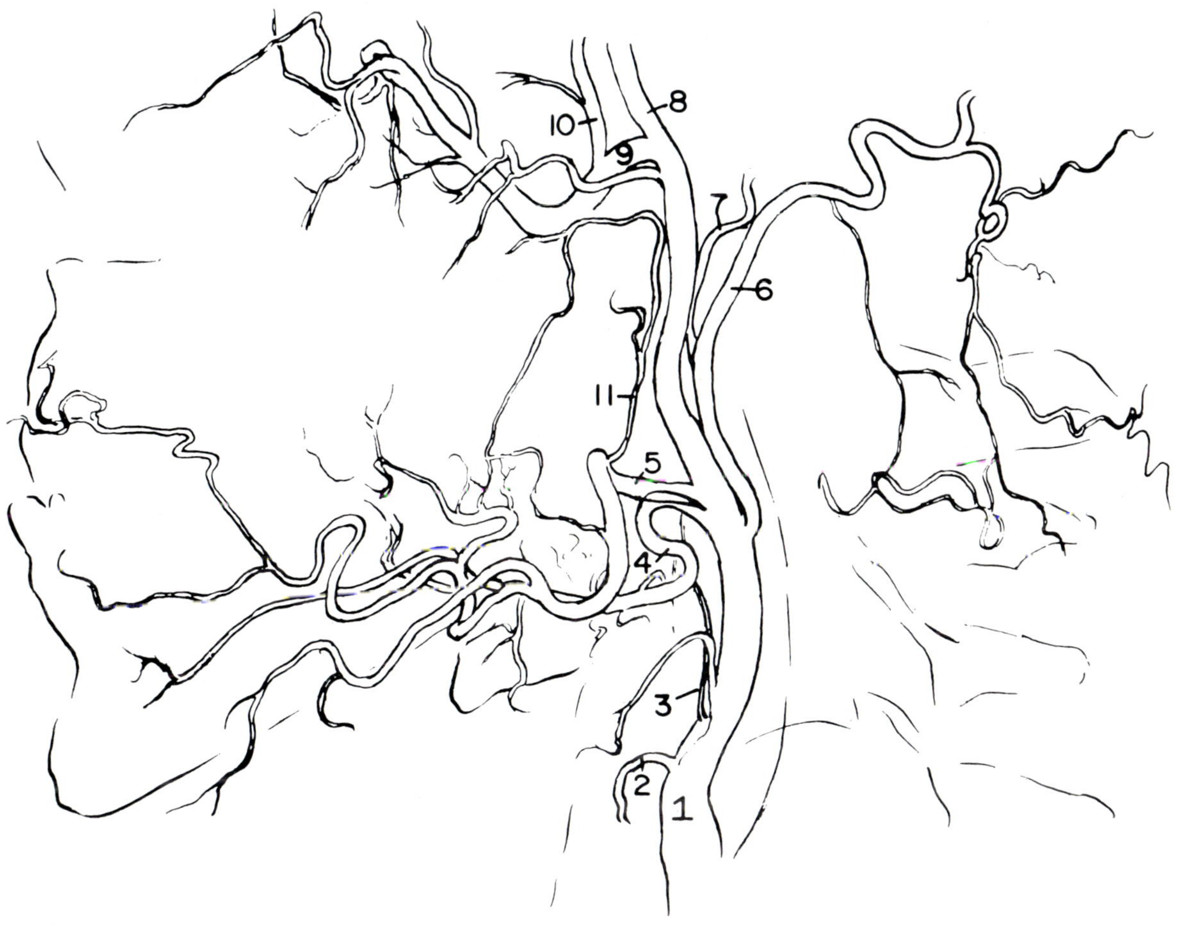

1. External carotid A.
2. Superior thyroid A.
3. Ascending pharyngeal A.
4. Lingular A.
5. External maxillary A.
6. Occipital A.
7. Posterior auricular A.
8. Superficial temporal A.
9. Internal maxillary A.
10. Middle meningeal A.
11. Ascending palatine A.

Vertebral Arteriogram

TRAY — Angiogram or Seldinger

NEEDLE — 16 or 18 gauge arteriographic or sheath (for left retrograde brachial) or headhunter catheter (Judkins design)

OPAQUE MEDIA — 60% meglumine diatrizoate or iothalamate

INJECTION RATE — 20 cc/sec for 2 to 2.5 sec with 1.2 sec x-ray delay (for left retrograde brachial) 4-6 cc total *by hand* if catheter is at vertebral origin and immediately withdraw catheter.

FILM RATE — 2/sec for 2 sec then 1/sec for 5 sec.

NOTES

If primary interest is the basilar artery, use lateral and submentovertex, otherwise use lateral and Towne's projection for visualization of the posterior fossa circulation.

The needle is inserted into the brachial artery just above the antecubital fossas as for right retrograde brachial. This study gives visualization of the posterior fossa circulation.

Manually compress the opposite subclavian to diminish dilution from the opposite vertebral and see the opposite posterior inferior cerebellar artery.

REFERENCES

1. Huang, Y. P., and Wolf, B. S.: The vein of the lateral recess of the fourth ventricle and its tributaries; roentgen appearance and anatomic relationships. Amer. J. Roentgenol., 101:1-21, Sept. 1967.
2. Mani, R. L., and Newton, T. H.: The superior cerebellar artery; arteriographic changes in the diagnosis of posterior fossa lesions. Radiology, 92:1281-1287, May 1969.
3. Pribram, H. F. W., Hudson, J. D., and Joynt, R. J.: Posterior fossa aneurysms presenting as mass lesions. Amer. J. Roentgenol., 105:334-340, Feb. 1969.
4. Scatliff, J. H., Kier, E. L., Zingesser, L. H., and Schechter, M. M.: Terminal basilar artery deformity secondary to suprasellar masses and third ventricular dilation. Amer. J. Roentgenol., 101:61-67, Sept. 1967.

NOTES

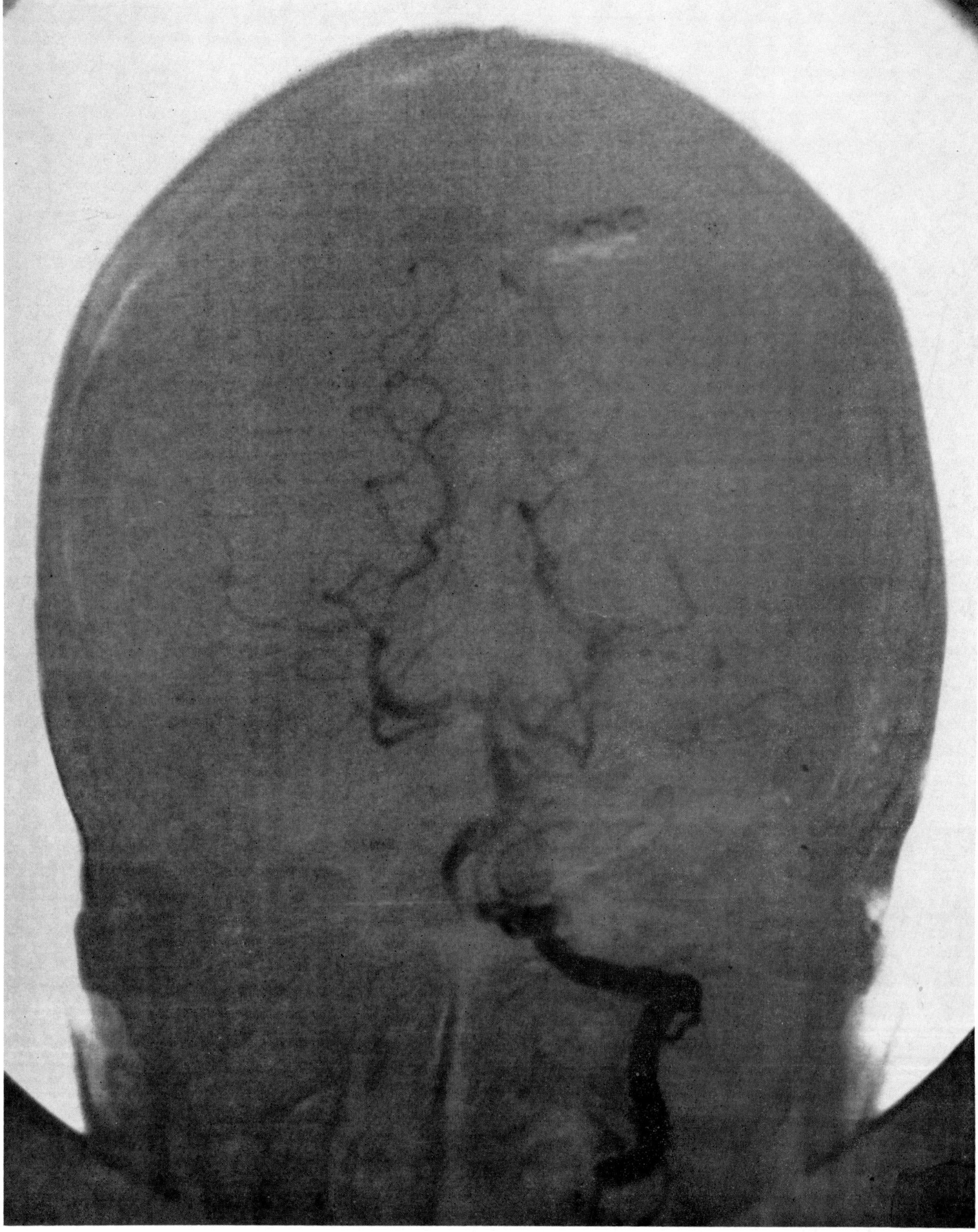

FIGURE 6. Vertebral Arteriogram (Anterior-posterior projection).

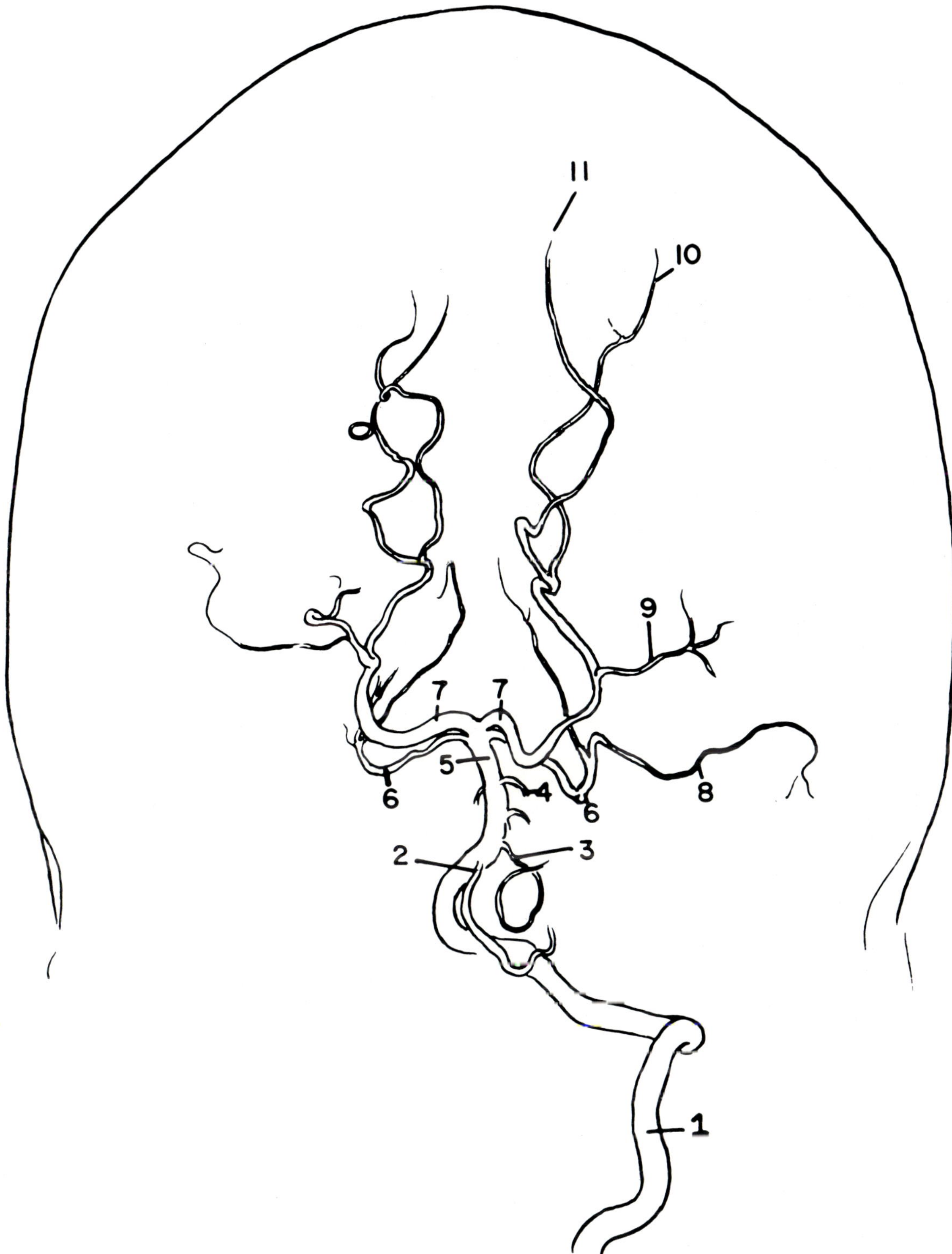

1. Vertebral A.
2. Posterior inferior cerebellar A.
3. Anterior inferior cerebellar A.
4. Pontine branches
5. Basilar A.
6. Superior cerebellar A.
7. Posterior cerebral A.
8. Marginal branch from superior cerebellar
9. Posterior temporal branch of posterior cerebral A.
10. Posterior occipital A.
11. Calcarine A.

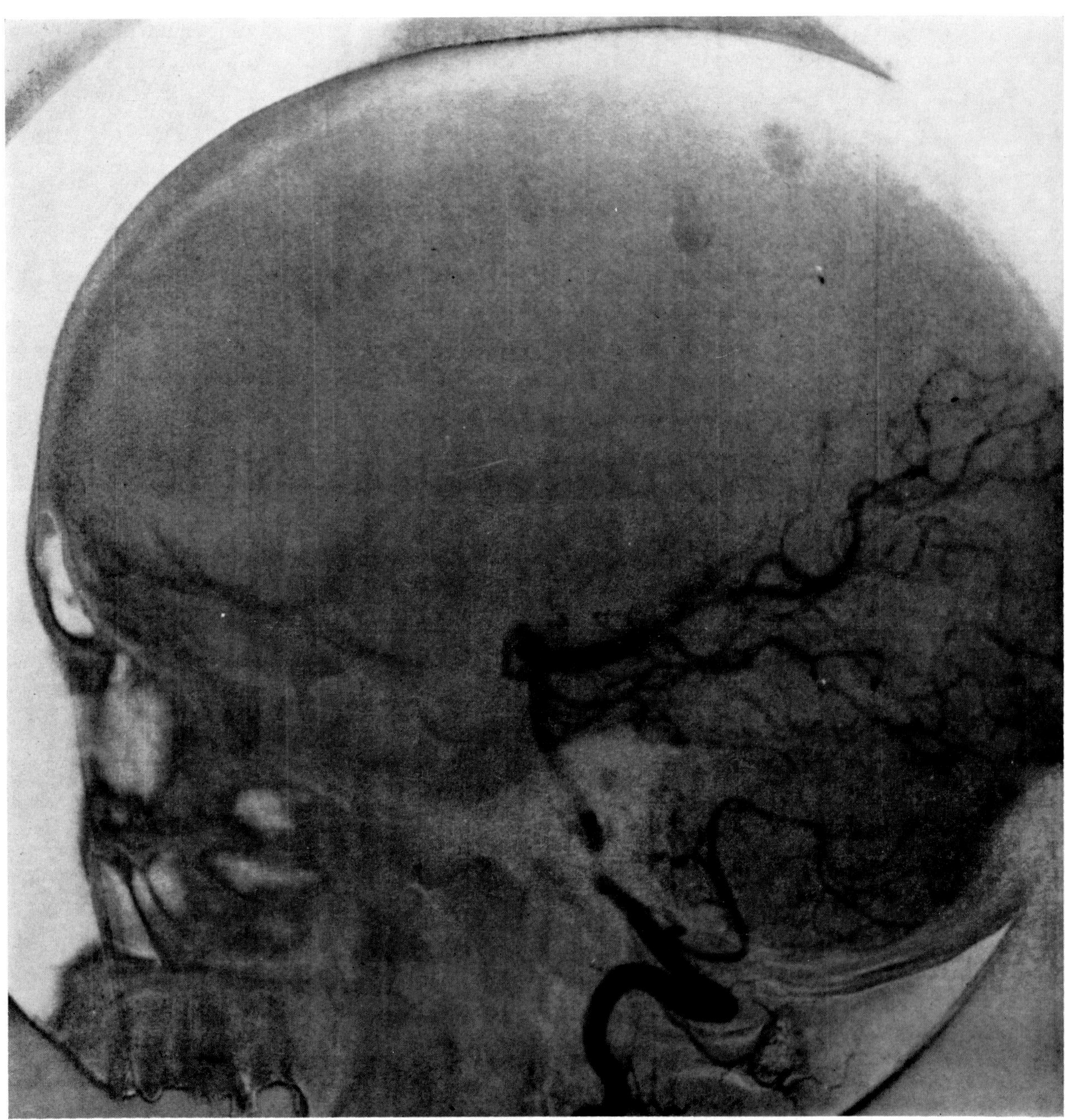

FIGURE 7. Vertebral Arteriogram (Lateral projection).

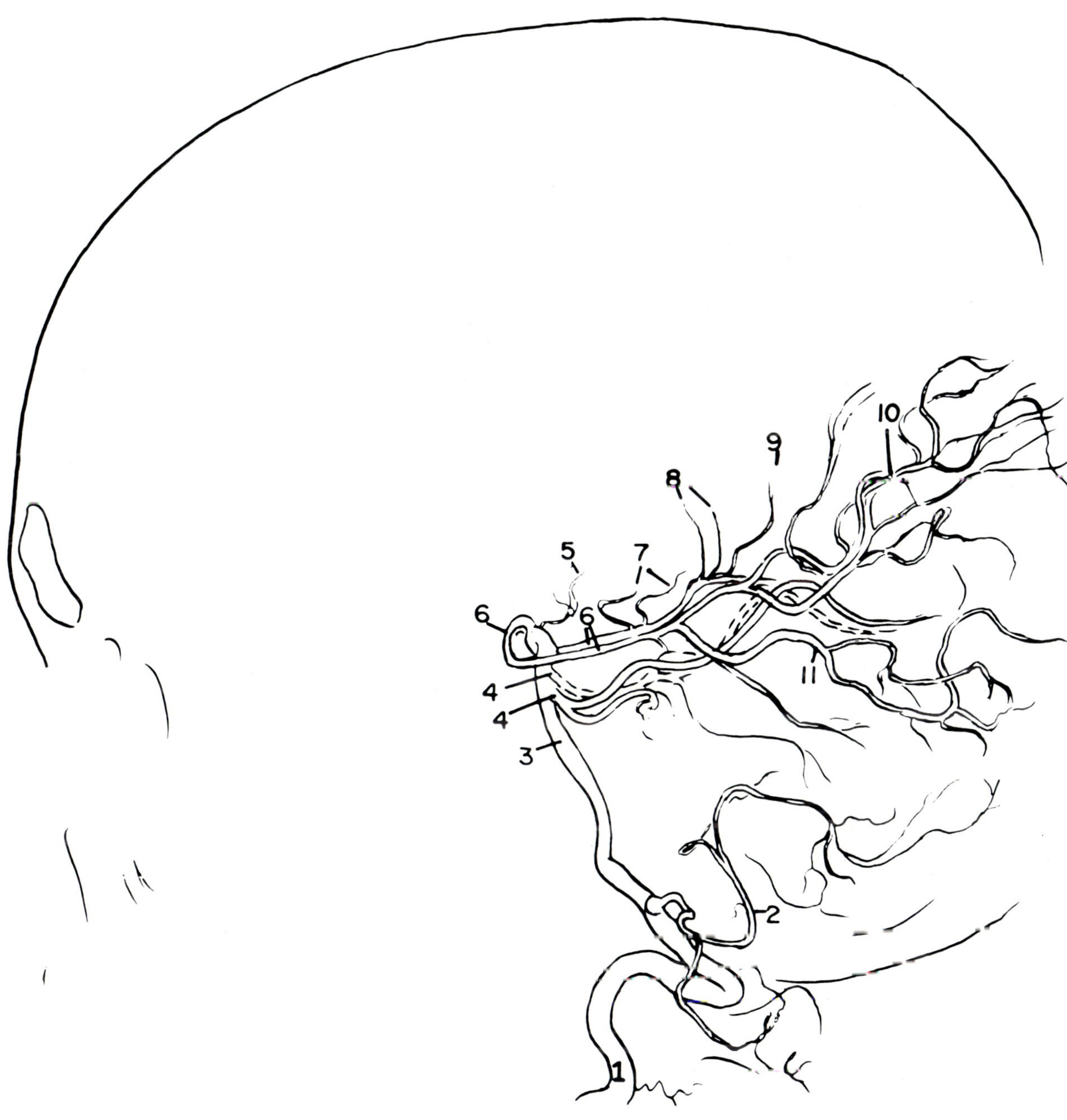

1. Vertebral A.
2. Posterior inferior cerebellar A.
3. Basilar A.
4. Superior cerebellar arteries
5. Thalamic arteries
6. Posterior cerebral arteries
7. Medial choroidal arteries
8. Lateral choroidal arteries
9. Dorsal callosal A.
10. Occipital arteries
11. Posterior temporal arteries

Right Retrograde Brachial Arteriogram

TRAY — Angiogram

NEEDLE — 16 gauge arteriographic or sheath needle and 12 P.E. 320 polyethylene (soft) connector.

OPAQUE MEDIA — 60% meglumine diatrizoate or iothalamate.

INJECTION RATE — 20 cc/sec for 2.25 sec with 1.5 sec x-ray delay (total 45cc)

FILM RATE — Routine 2/sec for 2 sec then 1/sec for 5 sec.

A-V malformation — 3/sec for 3 sec then 1/sec for 4 sec.

The filming sequence should be delayed approximately 1.5 sec relative to the beginning of injection. (variable with changer type.)

With increased intracranial pressure the filming sequence should be extended to cover 10 to 12 seconds.

NOTES

The brachial artery is punctured just above the antecubital fossa and the needle threaded into the arterial lumen while maintaining a good arterial flow. Injection and filming are done as described above. The needle and tubing, which connects the needle to the injector, must be secured to the patient's arm to prevent the needle from being jerked from the artery at the end of the injection. The stylet is replaced in the needle while the films are checked.

If several attempts at arterial puncture are unsuccessful, a cutdown with direct visualization of the artery during puncture may be done. The artery and tubing must still be secured to the arm even though a tie is placed around the artery and needle. The stylet is placed in the needle while the films are checked. It is usually necessary to repair the artery following the procedure because adequate hemostasis is difficult to obtain following interruption of the subcutaneous tissues.

For pediatric cases, use an 18 gauge angiographic or sheath needle and an injection rate of 20-30 cc by hand. Delay film sequence 0.9 sec and film at 2 to 3/sec for 3 sec then 1/sec for 3 sec. (To be used in the normal rapid flow dynamics of an infant or child). With high intracranial pressure, use adult sequence.

REFERENCES

1. Baird, R. M., Lapayowker, M. S., Murtagh, F., and Scott, M.: Percutaneous retrograde brachial arteriography; a nonoperative noncatheter technique. Amer. J. Roentgenol., 94:19-29, May 1965.
2. Boulos, R. S., Gilroy, J., and Meyer, J. S.: Technique of cerebral angiography in children. Amer. J. Roentgenol., 101:121-127, Sept. 1967.
3. Kuhn, R. A.: Brachial cerebral angiography. J. Neurosurg., 17:955-971, 1960.
4. Lindgren, E.: Another method of vertebral angiography. Acta Radiologica, 46:257-261, July-Aug. 1956.
5. Marshall, T. R., and Ling, J. T.: Direct percuaneous noncatheter left and right brachial angiography; (left panarteriography—right cerebral angiography). Radiology, 80:258-260. Feb. 1963.
6. Marshall, T. R., Ling, J. T., and Gonzalez, R.: Additional experiences with direct percutaneous noncatheter brachial angiography—Left panarteriography—Right cerebral angiography. Radiology, 81:568-575, Oct. 1963.

NOTES

THORAX

Thoracic Aortogram

TRAY — *S*eldinger arteriogram
CATHETER — #8 single curve (125 cm)
OPAQUE MEDIA — 76% meglumine and sodium diatrizoate
INJECTION RATE — 25 cc/sec for 2 sec (total 50 cc)
FILM RATE — 2/sec for 4 sec then 1/sec for 3 sec
NOTES

In positioning for the transverse portion of the arch and the origin of the brachio-cephalics, use the right posterior oblique position. For the ascending and descending aorta, the biplane A-P and lateral projection are preferable.

In dissecting aneurysms, identification of the point of entry into the false channel and the re-entry into the aorta are important for planning therapy. The femoral approach is preferred with the initial injection into the proximal ascending aorta where feasible.

REFERENCES

1. Hynes, D. M., and Grainger, R. G.: The angiographic demonstration of coarctation of the arota and similar anomalies. Clin. Radiology, 19:438-456, 1968.
2. Kirschner, L. P., Twigg, H. L., Conrad, P. W., and Hufnagel, C.: Retrograde catheter aortography in dissecting aortic aneurysms. Amer. J. Roentgenol., 102:349-353, Feb. 1968.
3. Lipchik, E. O., and Robinson, K. E.: Acute traumatic rupture of the thoracic aorta. Amer. J. Roentgenol., 104:408-412, Oct. 1968.
4. Shuford, W. H., Sybers, R. G., and Weens, H. S.: Problems in the aortographic diagnosis of dissecting aneurysm of the aorta. New Eng. J. Med., 280:225-231, Jan. 1969.
5. Stein, H. L., and Steinberg, I.: Selective aortography, the definitive technique for diagnosis of dissecting aneurysms of the aorta. Amer. J. Roentgenol., 102:333-348, Feb. 1968.

NOTES

Arch Study for Stroke Work-Up

TRAY — Seldinger Tray

CATHETER — #8 single curve (100 cm) with end and side holes
#7 headhunter (Judkins design) (100 cm) for selectives, if needed.

OPAQUE MEDIA — 76% meglumine and sodium diatrizoate for arch.
60% megulmine diatrizoate or iothalamate for selectives.

INJECTION RATE — Arch — 20 to 25 cc/sec for 2 sec
Innominate — 10-12 cc/sec for 2 sec
Left (or right) common carotid — 8 to 10 cc/sec for 1 sec
Left subclavian — 10 to 12 cc/sec for 2 sec
Selective vertebral — 2 to 3 cc/sec for 2 sec by hand (according to size and flow rate).
Remove catheter promptly.

FILM RATE — Arch — 2/sec for 4 sec with catheter 4cm above valve.
Selectives — 2/sec for 3 sec then 1/sec for 4 sec
Probable steal — 2/sec for 3 sec and 1/sec for 5 sec or cine.

POSITION — Arch RPO-biplane (AP upper chest and horizontal beam lateral neck).
Selectives routine cerebral position (angled AP and lateral).

NOTES

A key-hole shaped diaphragm is of value if filming the head and neck in the lateral projection.

REFERENCES

1. Amplatz, K. Resch, J., and Hilal, S.: A catheter approach for cerebral angiography. Radiology, 81: 576-583, Oct. 1963.
2. Cronqvist, S.: Total angiography in evaluation of cerebrovascular disease: a correlative study of aorto-cervical and selective cerebral angiography. Brit. J. Radiology, 39:805-810, Nov. 1966.
3. Hinck, V. C., Judkins, M. P., and Paxton, H. D.: Simplified selective femorocerebral angiography. Radiology, 89:1048-1052, Dec. 1967.
4. Janeway, R.: Current Techniques for Aortocranial Angiography. In: *Special Techniques for Neurological* Diagnosis, edited by James F. Toole. Philadelphia, Davis, 1969, ch. 7, pp. 139-181.
5. Poser, C. M., Zosa, A. M., Gomez, A. J., and Hardin, C. A.: Cervicocephalic angiography for cerebrovascular insufficiency. Acta Neurol. Scand., 40:321-336, 1964.
6. Weibel, J., and Fields, W. S.: Angiography of the posterior cervicocranial circulation. Amer. J. Roentgenol., 98:660-671, Nov. 1966.

NOTES

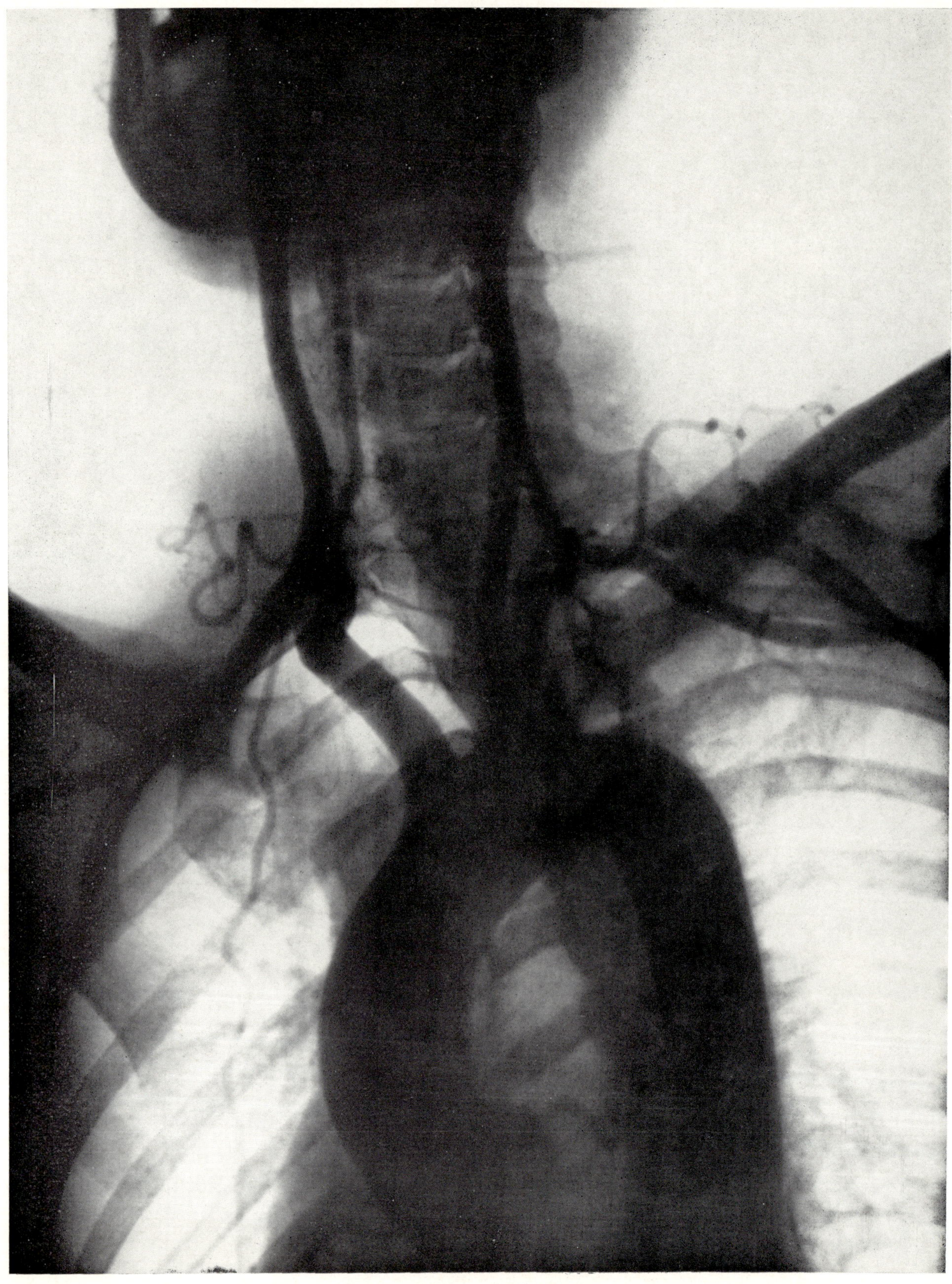

FIGURE 8. Thoracic Aortogram.

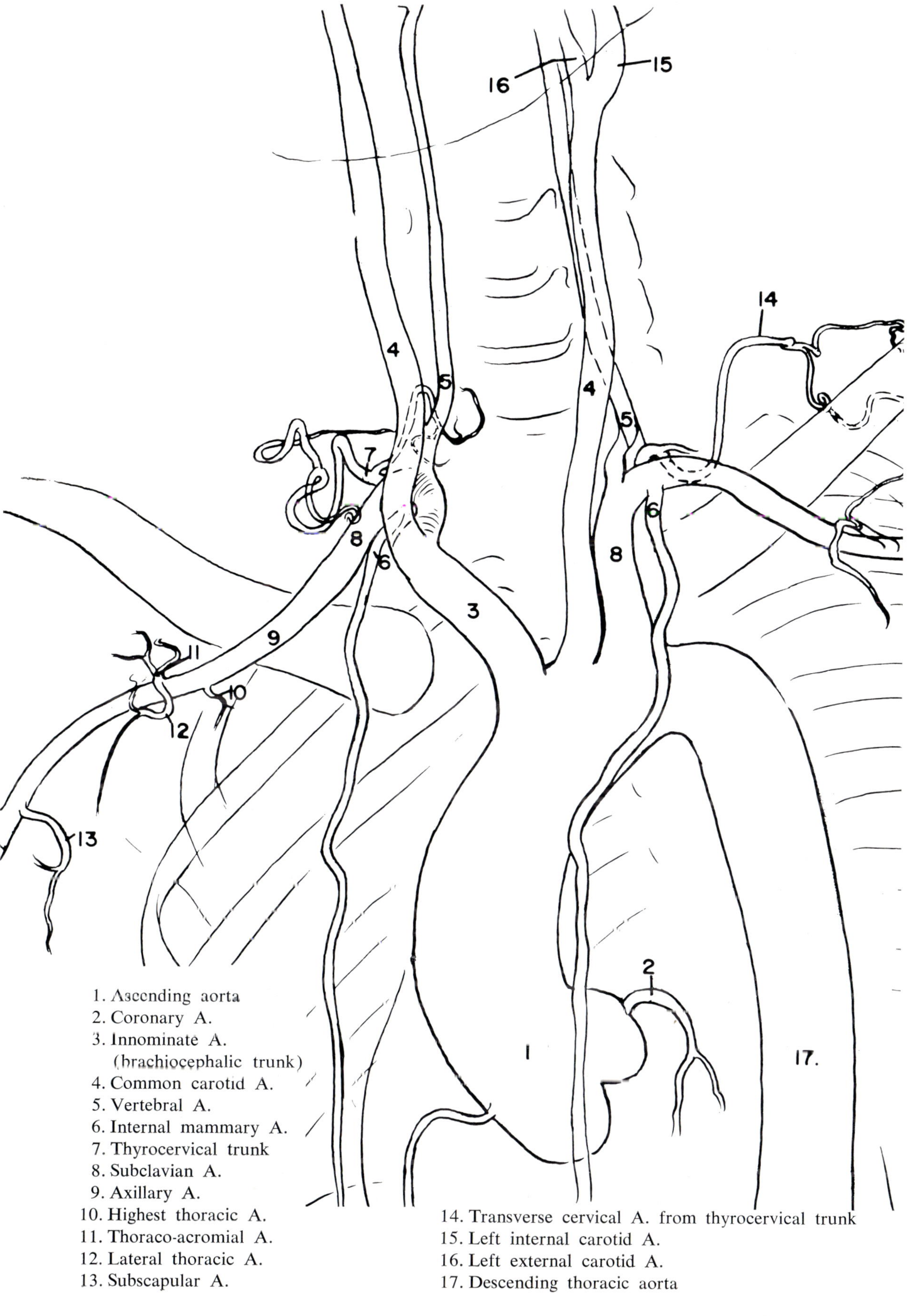

1. Ascending aorta
2. Coronary A.
3. Innominate A. (brachiocephalic trunk)
4. Common carotid A.
5. Vertebral A.
6. Internal mammary A.
7. Thyrocervical trunk
8. Subclavian A.
9. Axillary A.
10. Highest thoracic A.
11. Thoraco-acromial A.
12. Lateral thoracic A.
13. Subscapular A.
14. Transverse cervical A. from thyrocervical trunk
15. Left internal carotid A.
16. Left external carotid A.
17. Descending thoracic aorta

Superior Vena Cavogram

EQUIPMENT — (2) 50 cc syringes
2 Venotubes
2 #19 scalp vein needles
2 bottles of D5 water or one bottle and Y set-up.

OPAQUE MEDIA — 60% meglumine diatrizoate or iothalamate, if obstruction is present.
76% meglumine diatrizoate if unobstructed.

INJECTION RATE — by hand

FILM RATE — 1/sec for 6 sec starting with 10 cc left to inject.

NOTES

Inject both antecubital veins (one for control if the other is asymptomatic).

Don't have the patient inspire or Valsalva preparatory to filming.

Film in expiration. Extend the filming sequence with gross obstruction.

Following filming, the venotubing is attached to the D5 H2O to "wash out" the venous system and keep the needles open while the films are being checked.

REFERENCES

1. Hayt, D. B.: Roentgenographic signs of thrombosis of the superior vena cava and tributaries in neoplastic disease. Amer. J. Roentgenol., 93:87-89, Jan. 1965.
2. Roberts, D. J., Dotter, C. T., and Steinberg, I.: Superior vena cava and innominate veins; angiocardiographic study. Amer. J. Roentgenol., 66:341-352, Sept. 1951.
3. Steinberg, I.: Dilatation of the hemiazygos veins in superior vena caval occlusion simulating mediastinal tumor. Amer. J. Roentgenol., 87:248-257, Feb. 1962.
4. Steinberg, I.: Angiographic features of primary venous obstruction of upper extremity; Paget-Von Schrötter syndrome. Amer. J. Roentgenol., 98:388-396, Oct. 1966.
5. Steinberg, I., and Finby, N.: Great vessel involvement in lung cancer: angiocardiographic report on 250 consecutive proved cases. Amer. J. Roentgenol., 81:807-818, May 1959.

NOTES

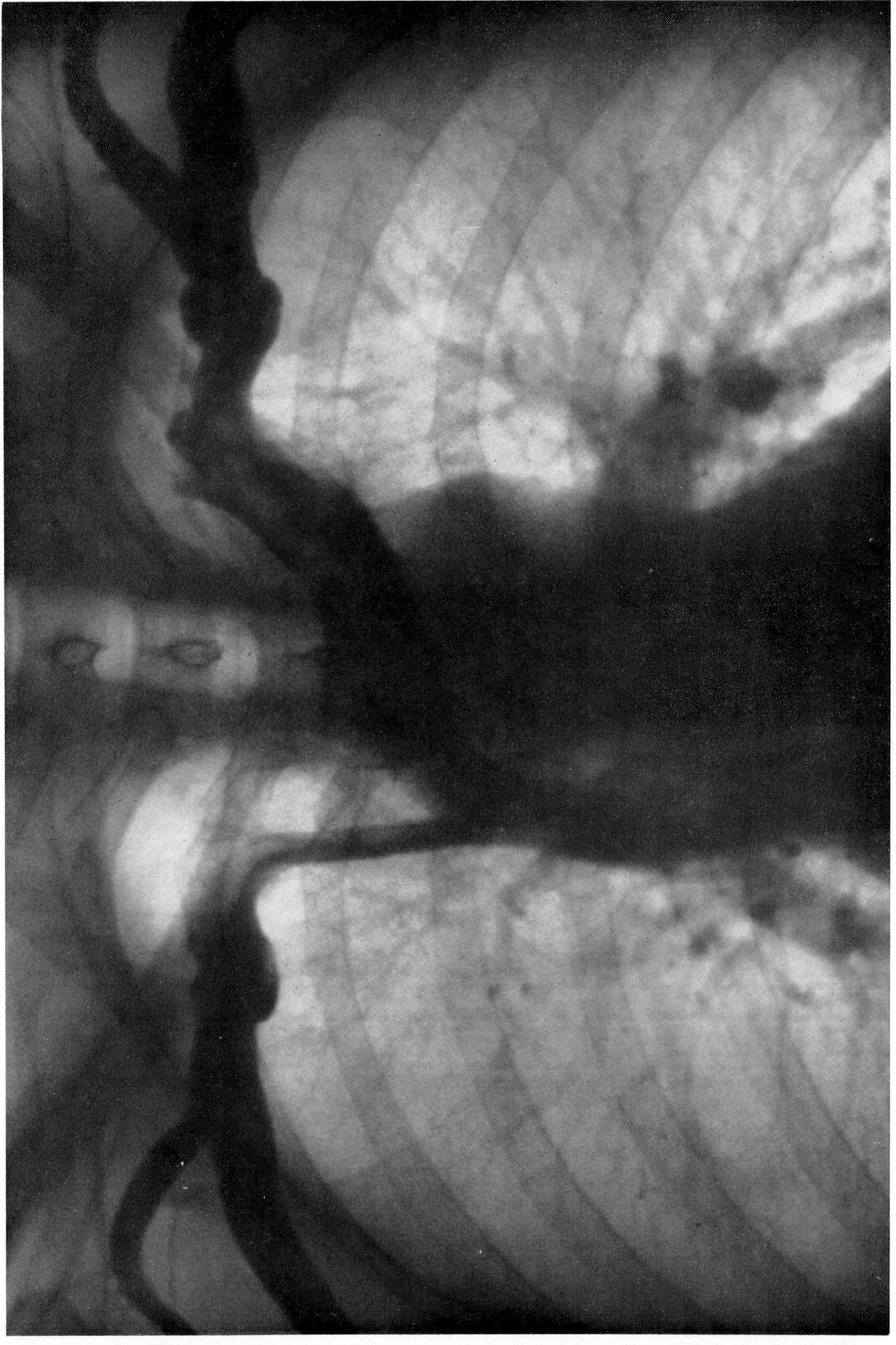

FIGURE 9. Superior Vena Cavogram.

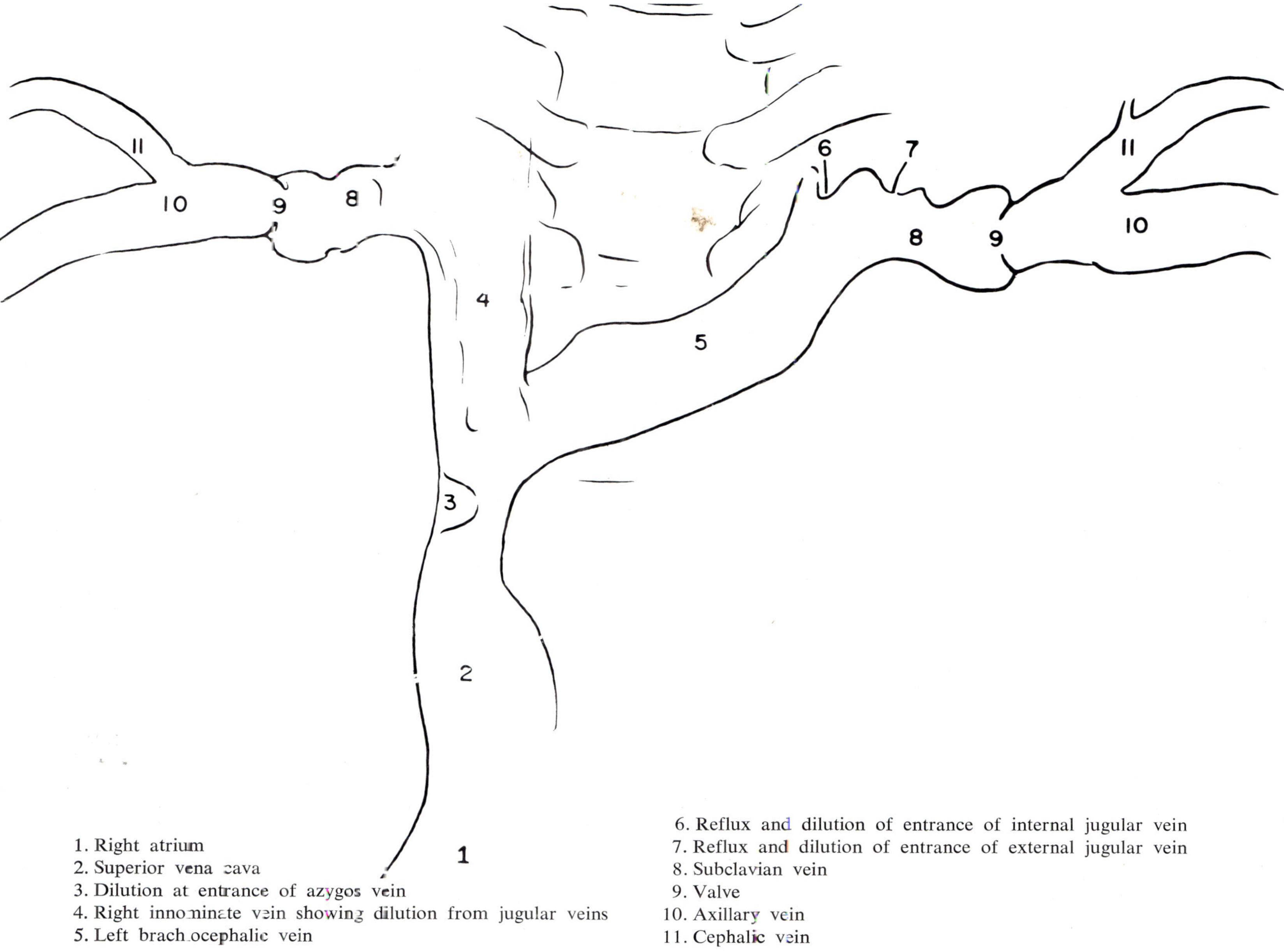
1. Right atrium
2. Superior vena cava
3. Dilution at entrance of azygos vein
4. Right innominate vein showing dilution from jugular veins
5. Left brachiocephalic vein
6. Reflux and dilution of entrance of internal jugular vein
7. Reflux and dilution of entrance of external jugular vein
8. Subclavian vein
9. Valve
10. Axillary vein
11. Cephalic vein

ABDOMEN

Aortogram

TRAY — Seldinger arteriogram (or translumbar)

CATHETER — #7 or #8 straight or single curve (60 to 80 cm) with *end and side* openings

OPAQUE MEDIA — 76% meglumine diatrizoate

For Survey:

INJECTION RATE — 20 cc/sec for 2 to 2.5 sec (total 40 to 50 cc)

FILM RATE — 2/sec for 3 sec and 1/sec for 4 sec

INJECTION SITE — At the middle of L-1

For Renals:

INJECTION RATE — 15 cc/sec for 3 sec
20 cc/sec for 2 sec

FILM RATE — 2/sec for 3 sec, and 1/sec for 4 sec

INJECTION SITE — ½ vertebral body *below* the highest renal artery.

NOTES

Technique — Perform injection and filming in deep inspiration (and with Valsalva maneuver if possible) to stretch out renals and temporarily lower cardiac output.

For hypertensive work-up, do aortogram *for renals* first. Follow with selectives as indicated. Film biplane with occlusive disease or aneurysm.

For renal cancer, do *survey* aortogram (to see metastases) after selective study of tumor.

For adrenal tumors, do *survey* aortogram first.

Translumbar: Check position of needle or sheath catheter with test dose and TV or Polaroid before giving definitive dose.

REFERENCES

1. Amplatz, K.: Translumbar catheterization of the abdominal aorta. Radiology, 81:927-931, Dec. 1963.
2. Bjorn-Hansen, R. W., and O'Brien, D. S.: Aortographic opacification of the gastric fundus simulating neoplasm. Amer. J. Roentgenol., 100:408-410, June 1967.
3. Love, L., and Braun, T.: Arteriography of peripheral vascular trauma. Amer. J. Roentgenol., 102: 431-440, Feb. 1968.
4. McDonald, P., and Hiller, H. G.: Angiography in abdominal tumours in childhood with particular reference to neuroblastoma and Wilms' tumour. Clin. Radiology, 19:1-18, Jan. 1968.
5. Muller, R. F., and Figley, M. M.: The arteries of the abdomen, pelvis, and thigh. I. Normal roentgenographic anatomy. II. Collateral circulation in obstructive arterial disease. Amer. J. Roentgenol., 77:296-311, Feb. 1957.
6. Nebesar, R. A., Fleischli, D. J., Pollard, J. J., and Griscom, N. T.: Arteriography in infants and children; with emphasis on the Seldinger technique and abdominal diseases. Amer. J. Roentgenol., 106:81-91, May 1969.
7. Palubinskas, A. J., Perloff, D., and Newton, T. H.: Fibromuscular hyperplasia; an arterial dysplasia of increasing clinical importance. Amer. J. Roentgenol., 98:907-913, Dec. 1966.
8. Roy, P.: Percutaneous catheterization via the axillary artery; an new approach to some technical roadblocks in selective arteriography. Amer. J. Roentgenol., 94:1-18, May 1965.
9. Steinberg, C. R., Archer, M., and Steinberg, I.: Measurement of the abdominal aorta after intravenous aortography in health and arteriosclerotic peripheral vascular disease. Amer. J. Roentgenol., 95:703-708, Nov. 1965.

NOTES

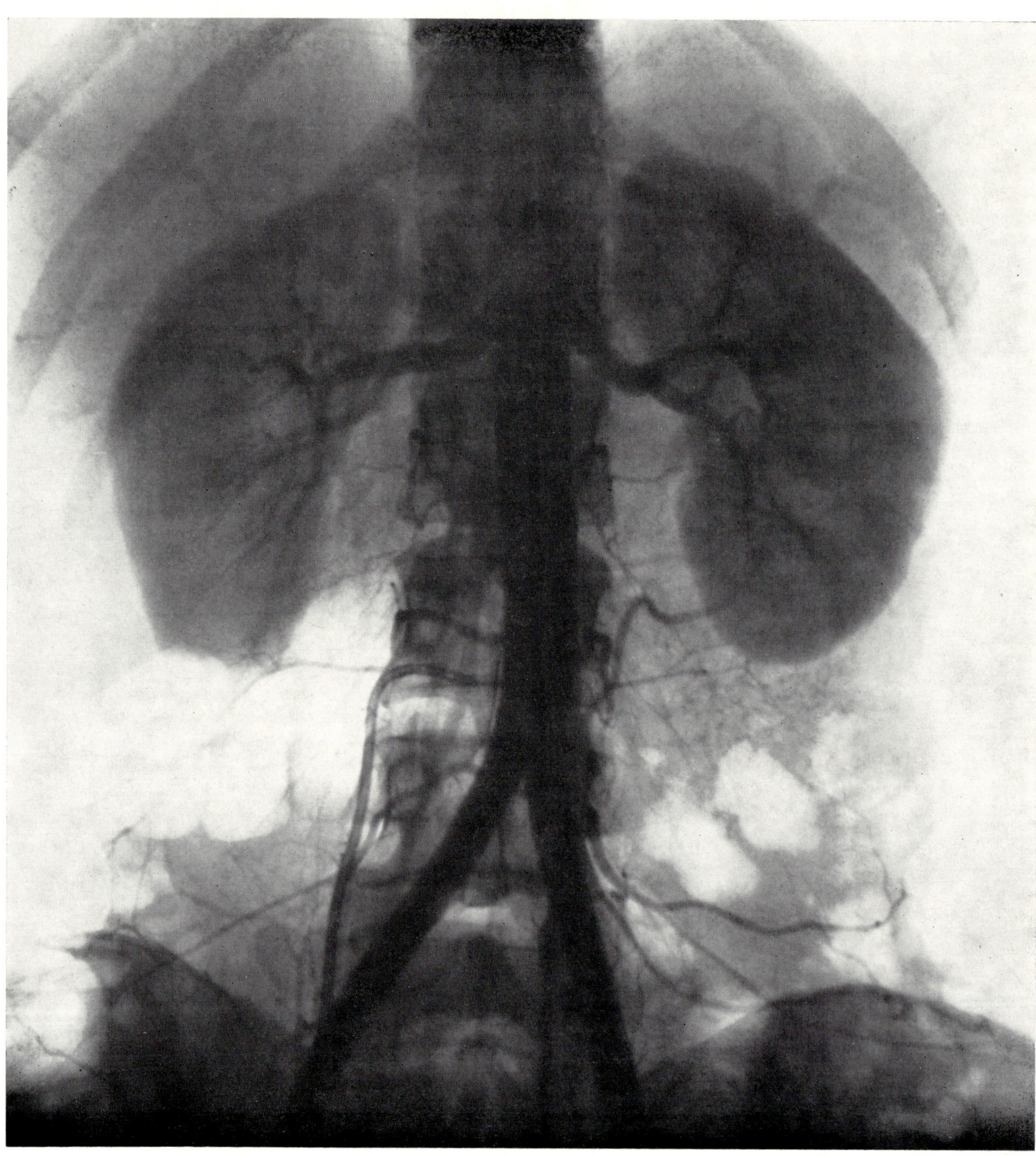

FIGURE 10. Abdominal Aortogram.

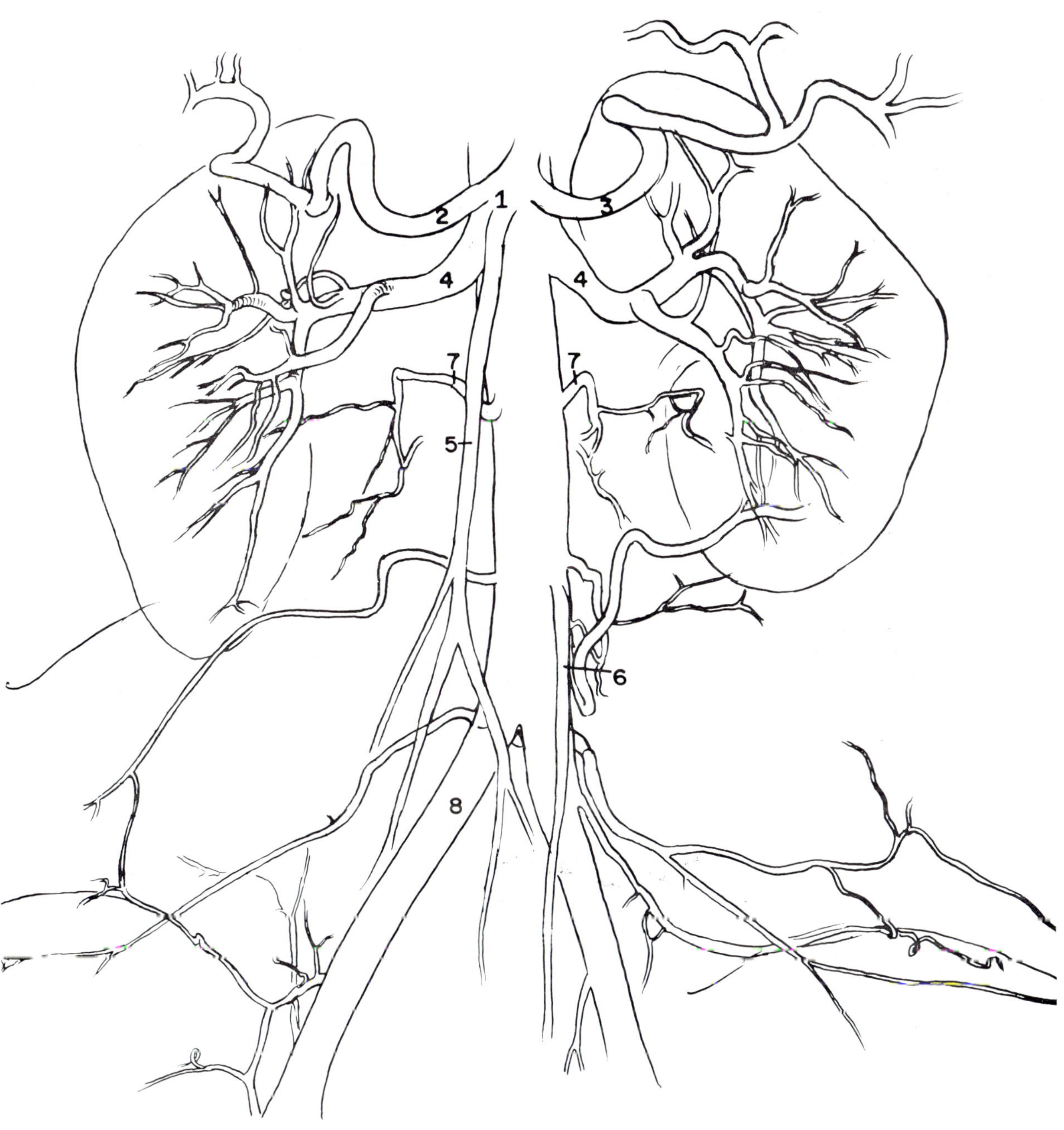

1. Aorta
2. Hepatic A.
3. Splenic A.
4. Renal A.
5. Superior mesenteric A.
6. Inferior mesenteric A.
7. Lumbars
8. Common iliac A.

Celiac Axis Arteriogram

TRAY — Seldinger arteriogram

CATHETER — #7 cobra 80 cm (Judkins design); #5 malleable end-opening (80 cm)

OPAQUE MEDIA — 76% meglumine diatrizoate

INJECTION RATE — Subselective 6 to 10 cc per sec for 5-10 sec (total 30-60 cc)

FILM RATE — Subselective hepatic for tumor (do mesenteric if right hepatic artery is not seen on celiac injection) 1/sec for 10 sec.
Subselective splenic for rupture 1/sec for 10 sec.
Pancreatic tumor (do splenic and pancreato-duodenal) 1/sec for 14 sec.
Twenty micrograms of adrenalin may help with questionable tumor patterns, but cut injection rate in half.
For bleeding 1/sec for 20 sec.
For occlusion or angina — biplane 1/sec for 7 sec (do at least one mesenteric in addition).

NOTES

The origin of the branches of the celiac arteries is variable with one of the more important variations being the origin of the right hepatic artery from the superior mensenteric artery. Knowledge of the origin of these vessels is important for the surgeon in planning perfusion of the liver in cases of metastatic disease. The celiac vessels originate superiorly from the aorta at the T-12 or L-1 area.

Origin of Hepatic Arteries: (10)

55% Right and left hepatic arteries from common hepatic artery from celiac.

10% Left hepatic arises from left gastric artery.

11% Right hepatic arises from superior mesenteric.

4.5% Common hepatic from superior mesenteric artery.

Small branch subselectives are more easily accomplished via the axillary route, with the double catheter technique or with specialized catheter manipulator devices.

REFERENCES

1. Alfidi, R. J., Rastogi, H., Buonocore, E., and Brown, C. H.: Hepatic arteriography. Radiology, 90:1136-1142, June 1968.
2. Boijsen, E.: Selective visceral angiography using a percutaneous axillary technique. Brit. J. Radiology, 39:414-421, June 1966.
3. Bron, K. M.: Selective visceral and total abdominal arteriography via the left axillary artery in the older age group. Amer. J. Roentgenol., 97:432-437, June 1966.
4. Bookstein, J., Reuter, S., and Martel, W.: Angiographic evaluation of pancreatic carcinoma. Radiology, 93:757-764, Oct. 1969.
5. Epstein, H. Y., Abrams, R. M., Beranbaum, E. R., and Localio, S. A.: Angiographic localization of insulinomas: high reported success rate and two additional cases. Ann. Surg., 169:349-354, Mar. 1969.
6. Kittredge, R. D., Colaiace, W. M., Kanick, V., and Finby, N.: The angiography of hemorrhage. Amer. J. Roentgenol., 107:181-190, Sept. 1969.
7. Lunderquist, A.: Angiography in carcinoma of the pancreas. Acta Radiologica: Suppl. 235, 1965.
8. Meaney, T. F., and Buonocore, E.: Arteriographic manifestations of pancreatic neoplasm. Amer. J. Roentgenol., 95:720-726, Nov. 1965.
9. Mikaelsson, C. G.: Polythene catheter of new shape for percutaneous selective catheterization. Acta Radiologica (Diag.), 3:581-591, Dec. 1965.

10. (Nebesar, R. A.), Kornblith, P. L., Pollard, J. J., Michels, N. A.: *Celiac and Superior Mesenteric Arteries: Correlation of Angiograms and Dissections.* Boston, Little, Brown, 1969.
11. Reuter, S. R.: Superselective pancreatic angiography. Radiology, 92:74-85, Jan. 1969.
12. Reuter, S. R., Redman, H. C., Miller, W. J., and Hoskins, P. A.: Gastric angiography. Radiology, 94:271-276, Feb. 1970.
13. Reuter, S. R., Redman, H. C., and Joseph, R. R.: Angiographic findings in pancreatitis. Amer. J. Roentgenol., 107:56-64, Sept. 1969.
14. Rösch, J., and Grollman, J. H.: Superselective arteriography in the diagnosis of abdominal pathology; technical considerations. Radiology, 92:1008-1013, Apr. 1969.
15. Rossi, P., and Ruzicka, F.: Differentiation of intrahepatic and extrahepatic masses by arteriography. Radiology, 93:771-780, Oct. 1969.
16. Ruzicka, F. F., and Rossi, P.: Arterial portography; patterns of venous flow. Radiology, 92:777-787, Mar. 1969.
17. Waldron, R. L., and Macken, K. L.: Celiac pancreatography. Presented at the Radiological Society of North America meeting, December, 1969.

NOTES

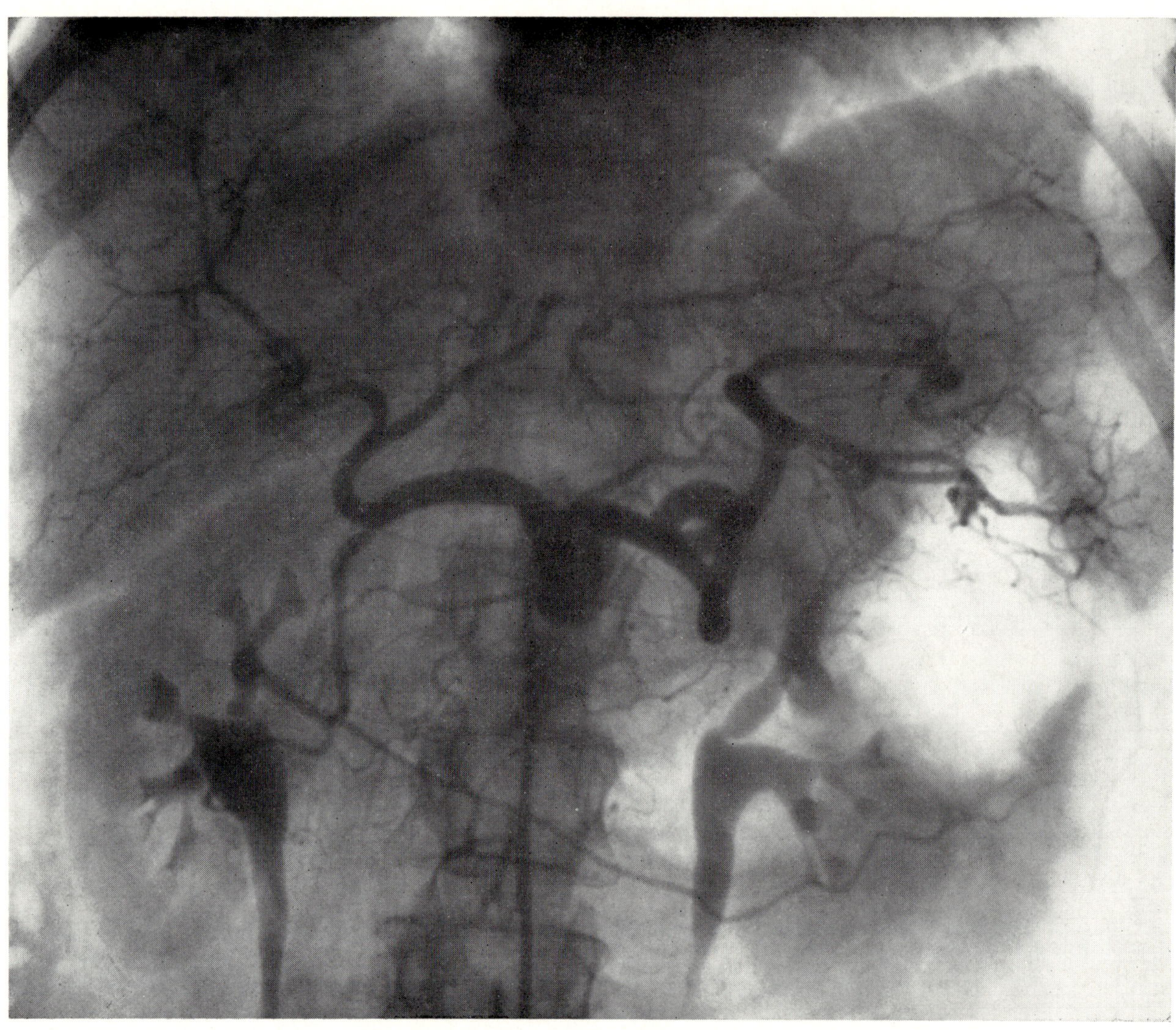

FIGURE 11. Celiac Arteriogram.

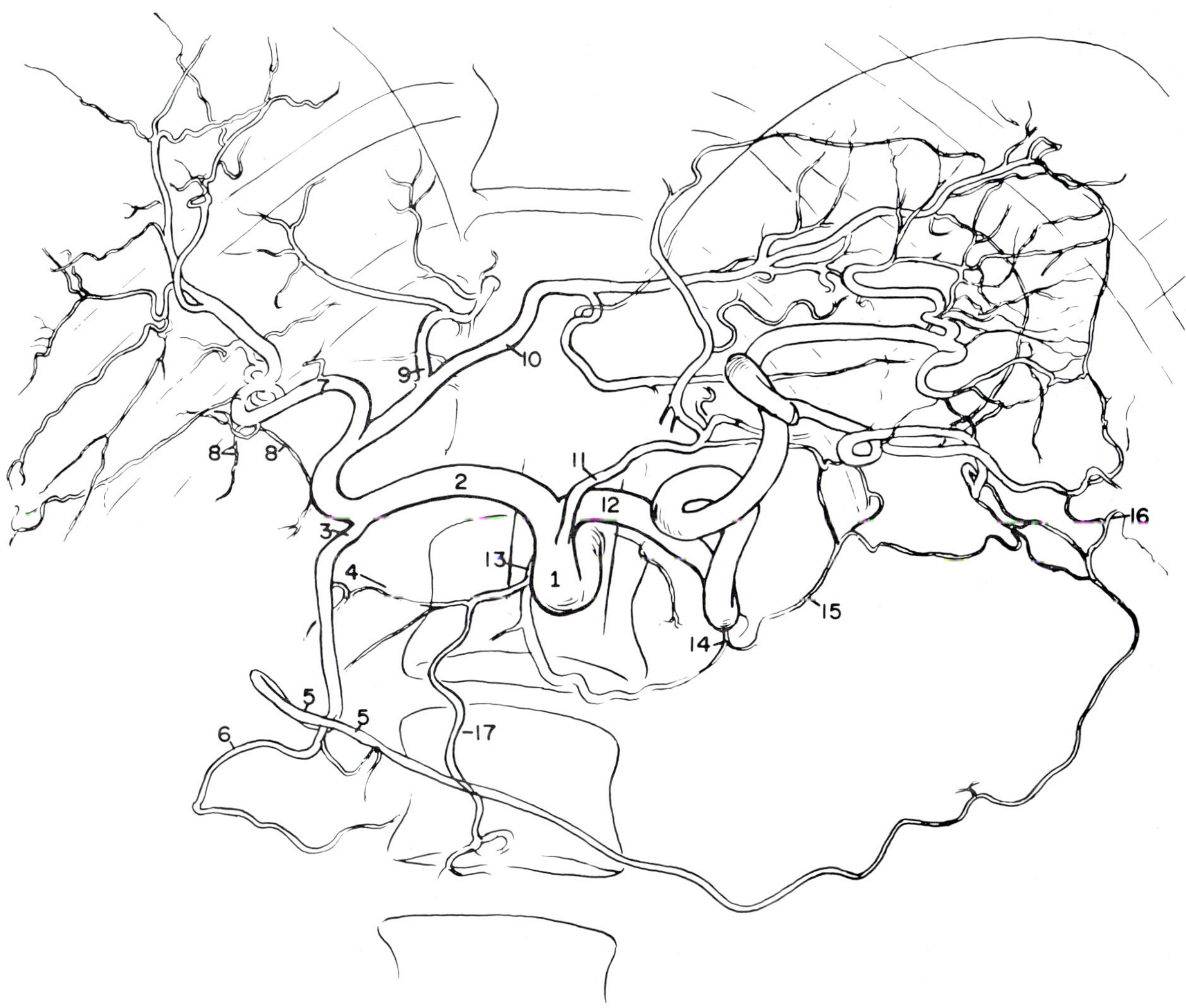

1. Celiac axis
2. Common hepatic A.
3. Gastroduodenal A.
4. Retroduodenal A. replacing posterior superior pancreaticoduodenal A
5. Right gastroepiploic A.
6. Anterior superior pancreaticoduodenal A.
7. Right hepatic A.
8. Branches of cystic A.
9. Middle hepatic A.
10. Left hepatic A.
11. Left gastric A.
12. Splenic A.
13. Dorsal pancreatic A.
14. Pancreatic magna A.
15. Transverse pancreatic A.
16. Left gastroepiploic A.
17. Anastomotic branch between celiac and superior mesenteric arteries

Superior Mesenteric Arteriogram

TRAY — Seldinger arteriogram
CATHETER — #7 cobra design (80 cm) Judkins design
OPAQUE MEDIA — 76% meglumine diatrizoate
INJECTION RATE — 5 to 8 cc/sec for 4-5 sec
FILM RATE — For occlusion or angina (biplane) 1.5 sec to 1/sec for 7 sec.
For bleeding, tumor, or varices (AP only) 1/sec for 20 sec
or 2/sec for 5 sec, 1/sec for 5 sec, 0.5/sec for 10 sec.

NOTES

The superior mesenteric artery originates from the abdominal aorta anteriorly about 1-2 cm below the celiac axis, and just above and medial to the left renal artery.

REFERENCES

1. Baum, S., Roy, R., Finkelstein, A. K., and Blakemore, W. S.: Clinical application of selective celiac and superior mesenteric arteriography. Radiology, 84:279-295, Feb. 1965.
2. Boijsen, E., and Reuter, S. R.: Mesenteric angiography in the evaluation of inflammatory and neoplastic disease of the intestine. Radiology, 87:1028-1036, Dec. 1966.
3. Bron, K. M., and Redman, H. C.: Splanchnic artery stenosis and occlusion. Radiology, 92:323-328, Feb. 1969.
4. Luderquist, A., Lunderquist, A., and Knutsson, H.: Angiography in Crohn's disease of the small bowel and colon. Amer. J. Roentgenol., 101:338-344, Oct. 1967.
5. Nebesar, R. A., Pollard, J. J., Edmunds, L. H., Jr., and McKhann, C. F.: Indications for selective celiac and superior mesenteric angiography; experience with 128 cases. Amer. J. Roentgenol., 92:1100-1109, Nov. 1962.
6. Reuter, S. R., and Boijsen, E.: Angiographic findings in two ileal carcinoid tumors. Radiology, 87: 836-840, Nov. 1966.
7. Sammons, B. P., Neal, M. P., Armstrong, R. H., and Hager, H. G.: Ten years experience with celiac and upper abdominal superior mesenteric arteriography. Amer. J. Roentgenol., 101:345-360, Oct. 1967.

NOTES

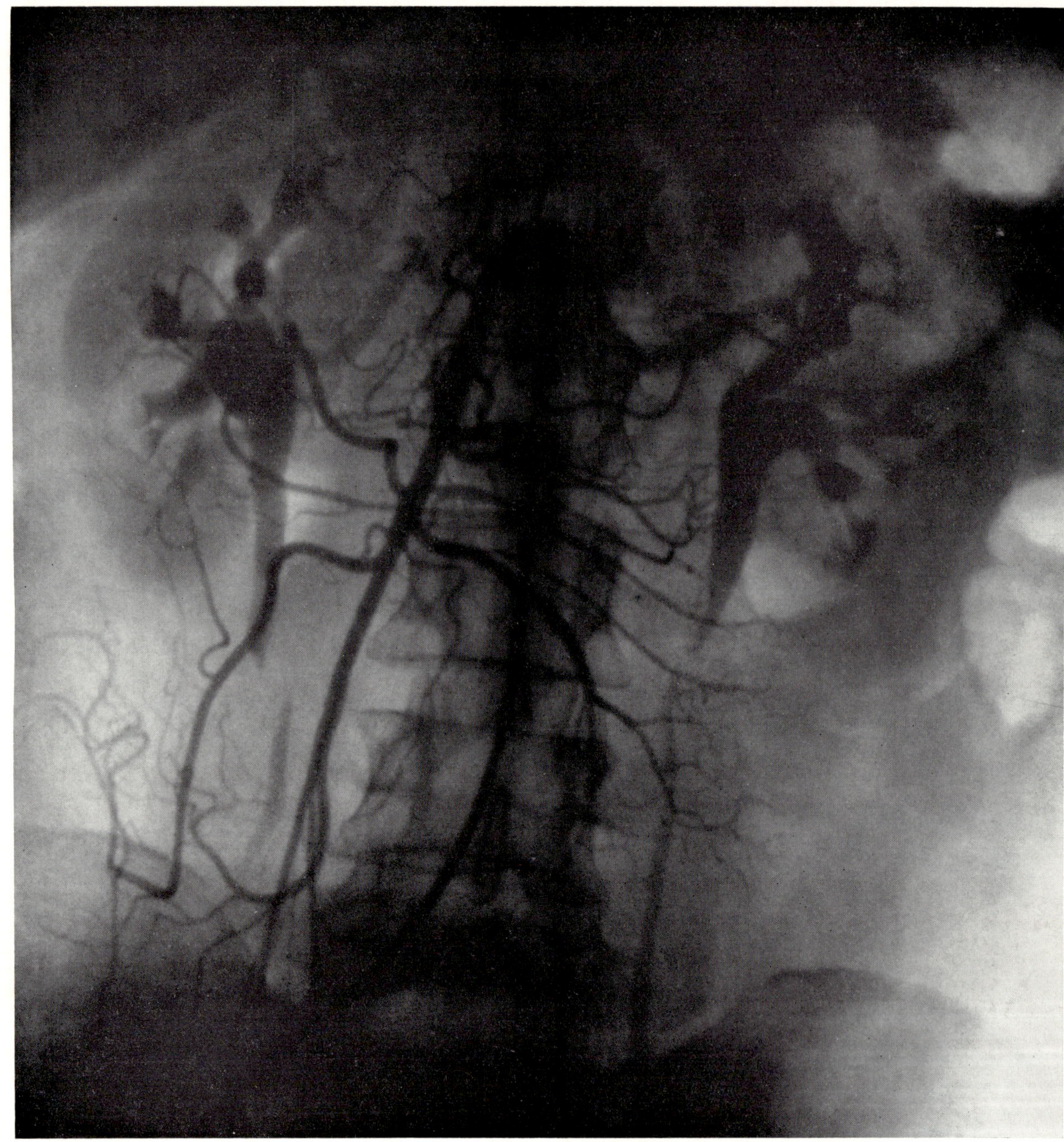

FIGURE 12. Superior Mesenteric Arteriogram.

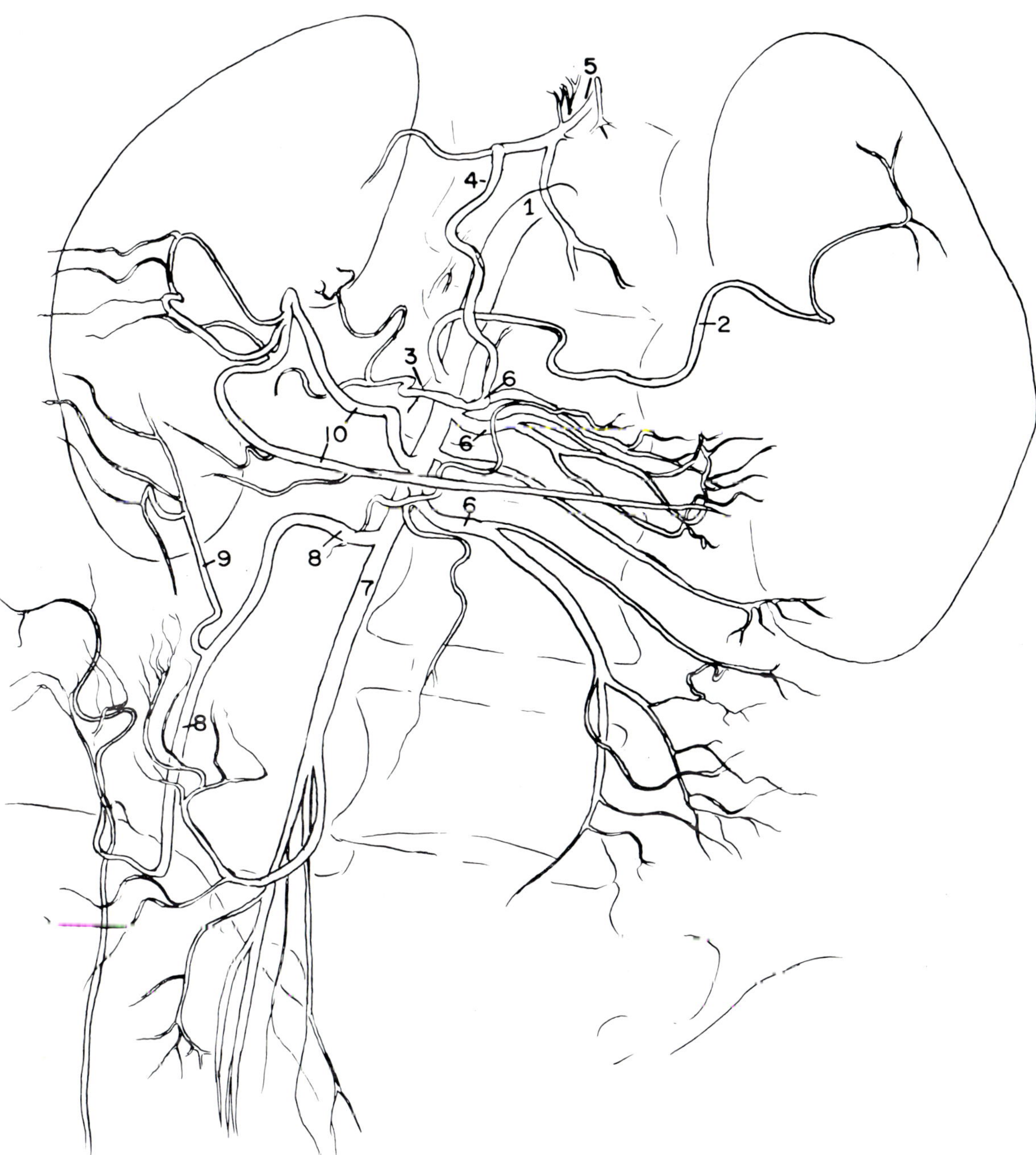

1. Superior mesenteric A.
2. Accessory middle colic A.
3. Inferior pancreaticoduodenal A.
4. Anastomotic branch between celiac and superior mesenteric arteries
5. Dorsal pancreatic A.
6. Jejunal A.
7. Ilial A.
8. Ilio colic A.
9. Accessory right colic A.
10. Right colic—middle colic common trunk

Inferior Mesenteric Arteriorgram

TRAY — Seldinger arteriogram
CATHETER — #7 cobra design (80 cm)
OPAQUE MEDIA — 60% or 76% meglumine iothalamate or diatrizoate.
INJECTION RATE — 4-5 cc/sec for 3-4 sec.
FILM RATE — Same as for superior mesenteric
NOTES

The inferior mesenteric arises from the anterior wall of the abdominal aorta at the level of L-3 or just above the aortic bifurcation.

REFERENCES

1. Kahn, P., and Abrams, H. L.: Inferior mesenteric arterial patterns; an angiographic study. Radiology, 82:429-442, Mar. 1964.
2. Ström, B. G., and Winberg, T.: Percutaneous selective angiography of the inferior mesenteric artery. Acta Radiologica, 57:401-410, Nov. 1962.

NOTES

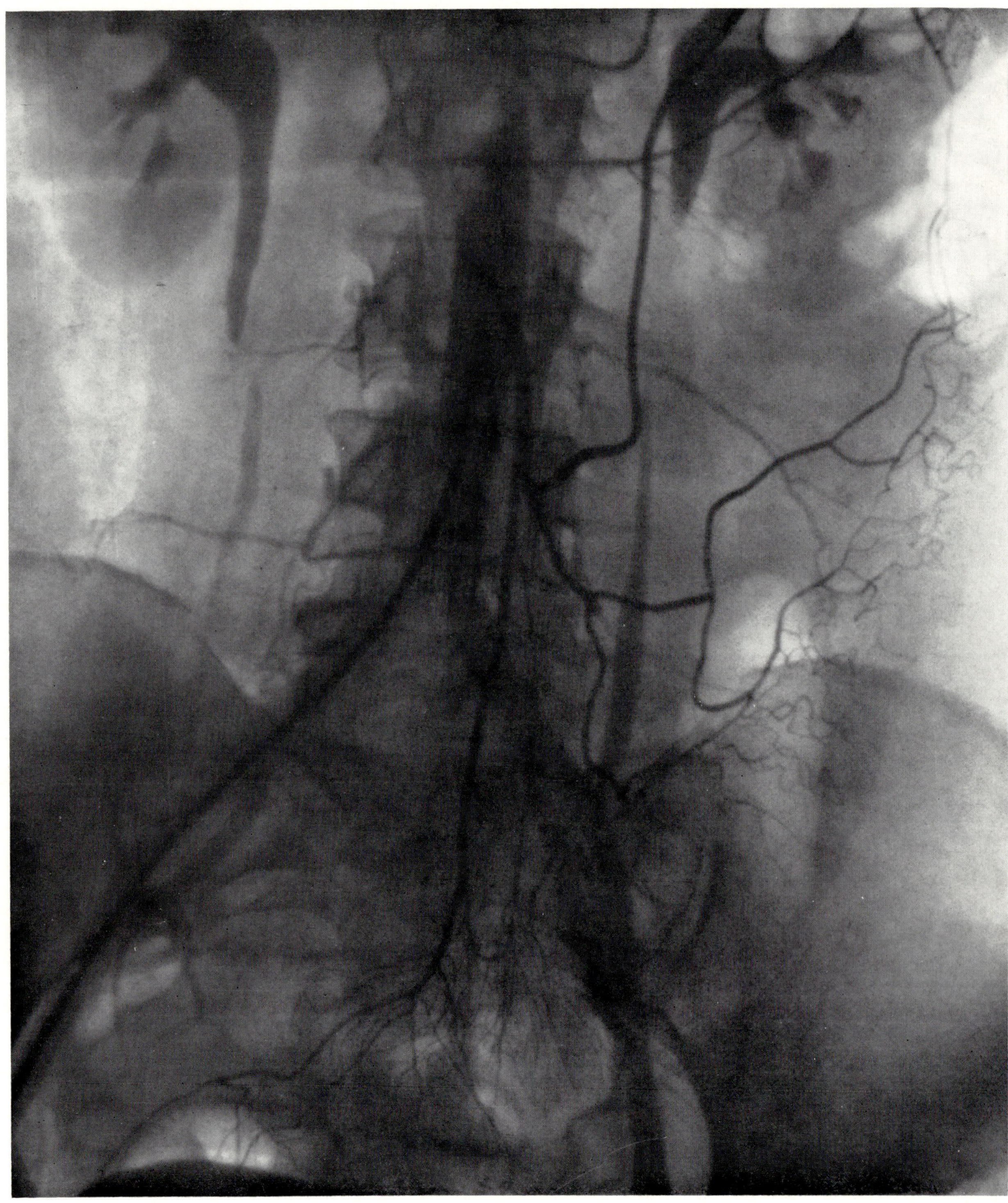

FIGURE 13. Inferior Mesenteric Arteriogram.

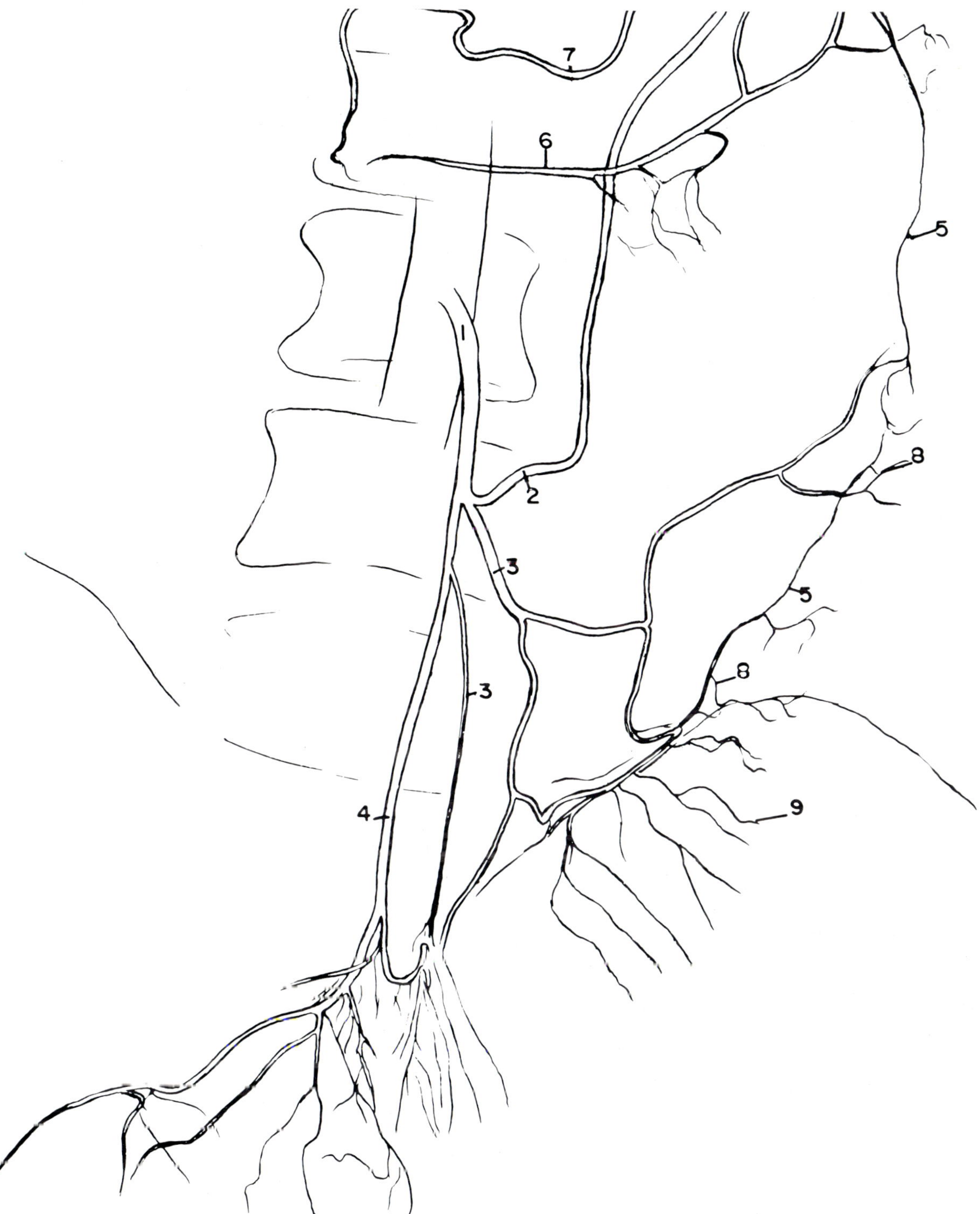

1. Inferior mesenteric
2. Left colic A.
3. Sigmoid A. (usually 3 in number)
4. Superior hemorrhoidal A.
5. Marginal A.
6. Middle colic from superior mesenteric*
7. Accessory middle colic A.
8. Vasa brevia (example)
9. Vasa longa (example)

*Griffith's point or the area of anastomosis between the middle colic and left colic is not on the film—but this area is usually at the splenic flexure.

Renal Arteriogram

TRAY — Seldinger arteriogram

CATHETER — #7 or #8 double curve (80 cm).

OPAQUE MEDIA — 60% or 76% meglumine diatrizoate or iothalamate.

INJECTION RATE — According to kidney and vessel size.
Normal single artery 4-8 cc/sec for 2 sec (less for multiple or low flow vessels)

FILM RATE — 1/sec for 7 sec
2/sec for 3 sec, 1/sec for 4 sec in tumor suspects.

NOTES

1. *Tumor Technique* — Overdose large renal cancers to see venous drainage and extend filming sequence to 10-12 sec.

Do survey aortogram and selective injections to see metastases in obvious renal cancer.

Consider adrenalin (10 micrograms) in equivocal abnormal vascular patterns. Normal renal vessels constrict whereas abnormal vessels as in renal carcinoma, hamartomas and certain inflammatory lesions do not.

Consider percutaneous puncture to verify "cysts."

Inferior venacavography and/or selective renal venography are usually needed with renal cancer.

2. *Anatomic Study Prior to Nephrotomy*. For avascular surgery for renal calculi (13). This allows labeling of anterior and posterior divisions of renal artery.

Selective A-P (1/7)

Stereo[A-P] (1/4) arterial phase only.

Oblique — same side down — arterial phase only.

In the straight AP, the arcuate arteries of the anterior (ventral) branches project nearer the free edge of the kidney than those of the posterior (dorsal) branches.

In the oblique view, the anterior arteries rotate laterally and the posterior arteries medially.

3. *Hypertensive Techniques* — "Renal aortogram" first (catheter tip just below highest renal.)

Selectives as needed.

Obliques may be needed to visualize the origin of the renal arteries. If the side opposite the kidney to be studied is obliqued downward, a posterolatral origin of the artery will be better visualized. The right renal artery, and less frequently the left renal artery, may arise close to the ventral midline of the aorta, and the side to be studied is then obliqued downward (RPO for right) to project the origin in profile (10).

Consider renal vein renins in stenoses or contracted kidneys with hypertension.

REFERENCES

1. Abrams, H. L.: The response of neoplastic renal vessels to epinephrine in man. Radiology, 82:217-224, Feb. 1964.
2. Becker, J. A., Fleming, R., Kanter, I., and Melicow, M.: Misleading appearances in renal angiography. Radiology, 88:691-700, Apr. 1967.
3. Boijsen, E.: Angiographic studies of the anatomy of single and multiple renal arteries. Acta Radiologica: Suppl. 183, 1959.

4. Caplan, L. H., Siegelman, S. S., and Bosnaik, M. A.: Angiography in inflammatory space-occupying lesions of the kidney. Radiology, 88:14-23, Jan. 1967.
5. Folin, J.: Angiography in Wilms' tumor. Acta Radiologica (Diag.), 8:201-208, May 1969.
6. Foster, R. S., Shuford, W. H., and Weens, H. S.: Selective renal arteriography in medial diseases of the kidney. Amer. J. Roentgenol., 95:291-308, Oct. 1965.
7. Khilnani, M. T., Abrams, R. M., and Beranbaum, E. R.: Angiographic features of hamartoma of the kidney; a case report. Radiology, 90:999-1000, May 1968.
8. March, T. L., and Halpern, M.: Renal vein thrombosis demonstrated by selective renal phlebography. Radiology, 81:958-962, Dec. 1963.
9. McDonald, P., and Hiller, H. G.: Angiography in abdominal tumours in childhood with particular reference to neuroblastoma and Wilms' tumour. Clin. Radiology, 19:1-18, Jan. 1968.
10. Ödman, P., and Ranniger, K.: The location of the renal arteries; an angiographic and postmortem study. Amer. J. Roentgenol., 104:283-288, Oct. 1968.
11. Palmisano, P.: Renal hamartoma (angiomyolipoma); is angiographic appearance and response to intra-arterial epinephrine. Radiology, 88:249-252, Feb. 1967.
12. Kincaid, Owings W., ed.: *Renal Angiography*. Chicago, Year Book Medical Publishers, 1966.
13. Smith, M. J. V., and Boyce, W. H.: Anatrophic nephrotomy and plastic calyrhaphy. J. Urol., 99: 521-527, May 1968.
14. Watson, R. C., Fleming, R. J., and Evans, J. A.: Arteriography in the diagnosis of renal carcinoma. Radiology, 91:888-897, Nov. 1968.

NOTES

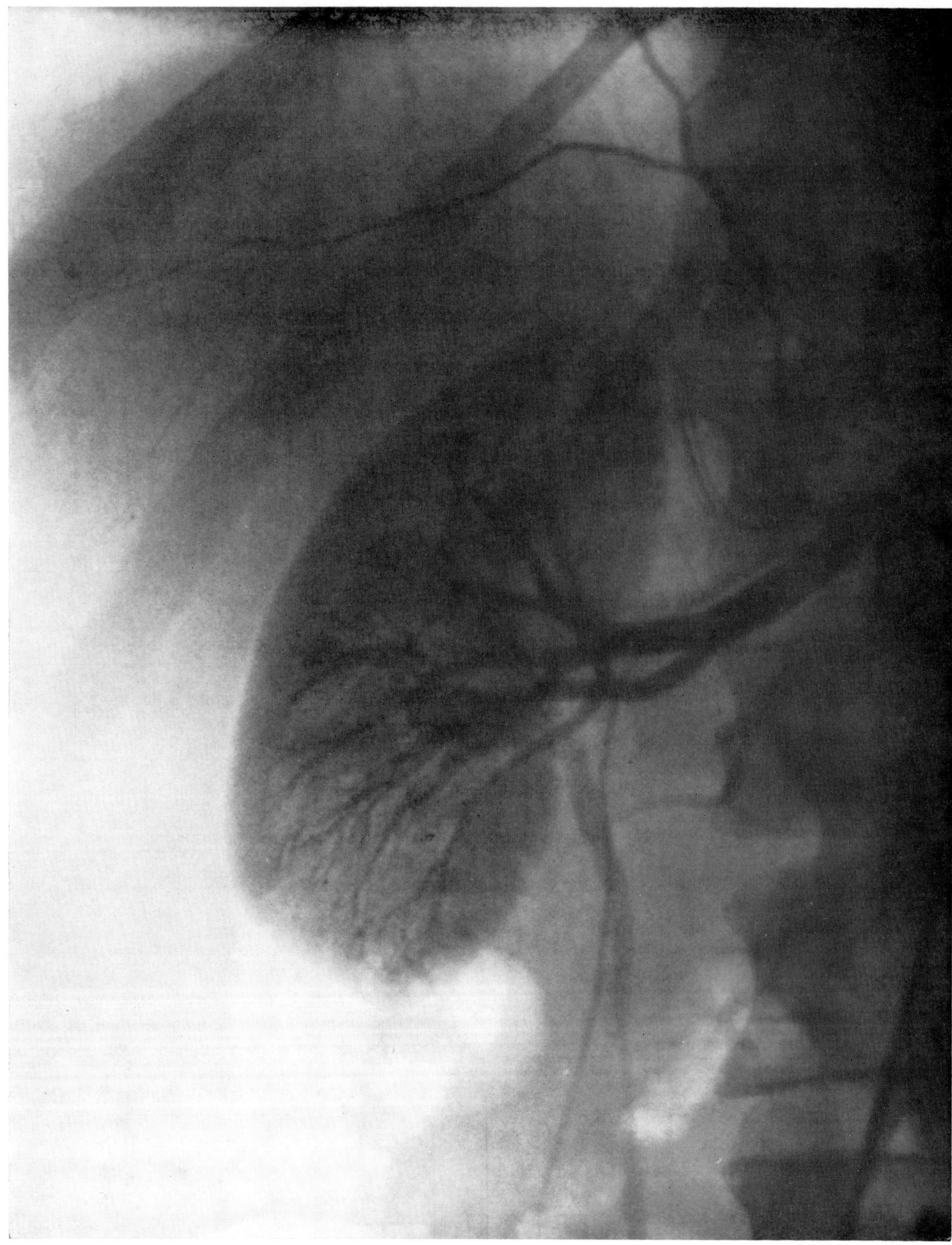

FIGURE 14. Renal Arteriogram.

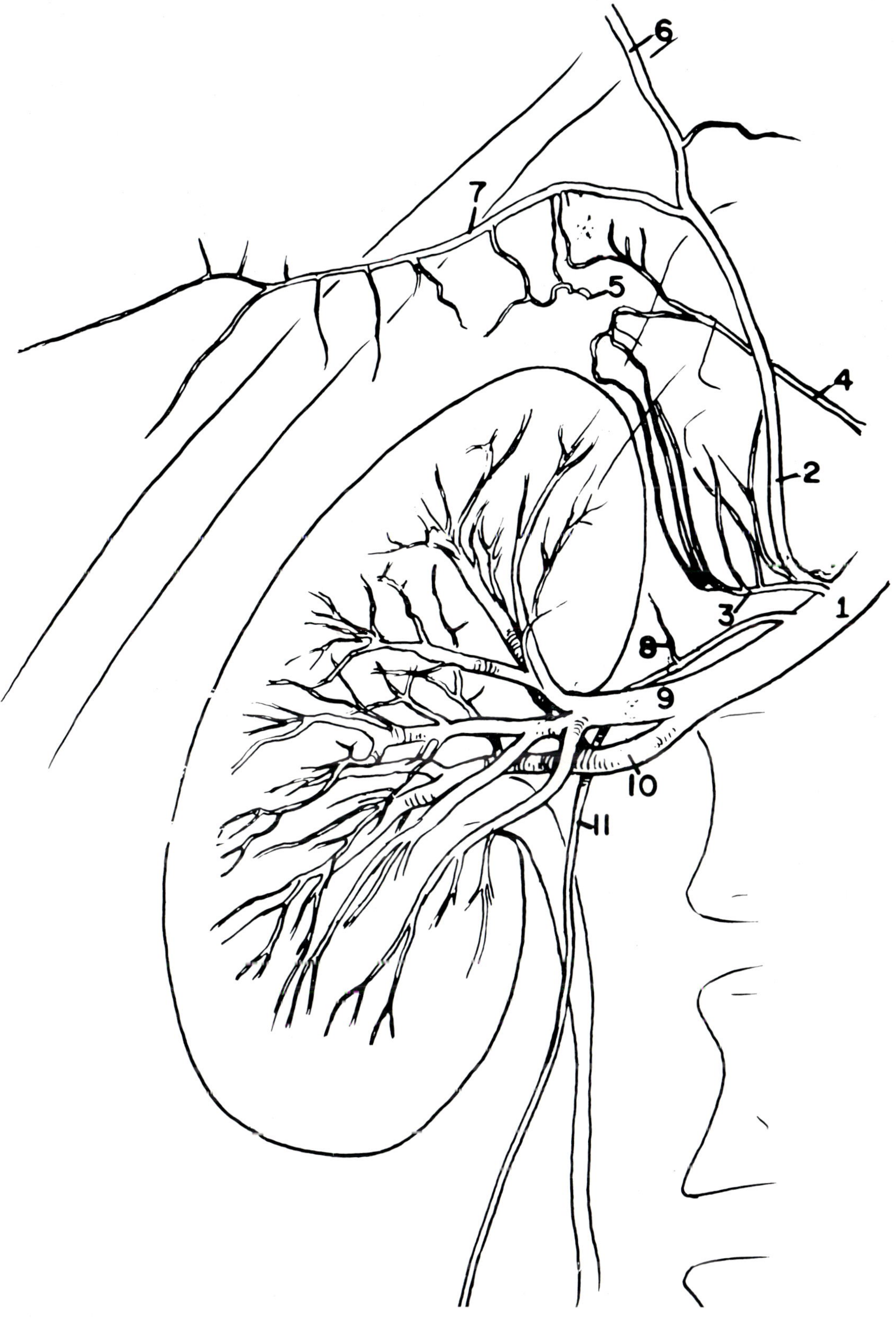

1. Renal A.
2. Inferior phrenic A.
3. Inferior adrenal arteries
4. Middle adrenal A.
5. Superior adrenal arteries
6. Anterior division of inferior phrenic A.
7. Posterior division of inferior phrenic A.
8. Capsular A. (from gonadal)
9. Ventral (anterior) branch of Renal A.
10. Dorsal (posterior) branch of Renal A.
11. Gonadal A.

Adrenal Arteriogram

TRAY — Seldinger Arteriogram

CATHETER — #7 or #8 single curve or straight catheter with side and end holes for aortogram.
#7 double curve (80 cm) for selective renal.
#5 malleable end opening (80 cm) for middle adrenal.

OPAQUE MEDIA — 76% meglumine diatrizoate

INJECTION RATE — Selective renals 2-3 cc/sec for 3 to 4 sec after 10 micrograms of adrenalin.
Selective "middle" and inferior phrenic by hand very gently 3 to 6 cc.
Celiac 3 cc/sec for 4 sec after 20 micrograms of adrenalin.

FILM RATE — 1/sec for 10 sec

NOTES

In pheochromocytoma suspects, have Regitine in a syringe ready for use, and intravenous fluids in place to provide a route for injection of Regitine.

Begin with a survey aortogram, then selective renals and middle adrenals and inferior phrenics. Adrenalin, 10 micrograms into the renal artery will increase the flow (relative) to the inferior adrenal artery. Adrenalin, 20 micrograms can be injected into celiac. One tenth of one cubic centimeter of the usual 1:1000 ampule diluted to 10 cc equals 10 micrograms per cc. Dilute the definitive adrenalin dose with 5 to 10 cc of saline prior to injecting the dose into the artery. Maximum pharmacologic effort is present within 15 seconds after infusion and diminishes over the next minute. Injection of only one source of adrenal blood supply may give a false impression of gland size by filling only a portion of it.

Inferior phrenic origin: Right: 46% aortic
9% right renal
Left: 52% celiac
Common trunk: 31%

REFERENCES

1. Alifidi, R. J., Gill, W. M., and Klein, H. J.: Arteriography of adrenal neoplasms. Amer. J. Roentgenol., 106:635-641, July 1969.
2. Kahn, P. C.: Selective angiography of the inferior phrenic arteries. Radiology, 88:1-8, Jan. 1967.
3. Kahn, P. C., and Nickrosz, L. V.: Selective angiography of the adrenal glands. Amer. J. Roentgenol., 101:739-749, Nov. 1967.
4. Lagergren, C.: Angiographic changes in the adrenal glands. Amer. J. Roentgenol., 101:732-738, Nov. 1967.
5. Lang, E. K.: The roentgenographic diagnosis of suprarenal masses. Radiology, 87:35-45, July 1966.
6. Lindvall, N., and Slezak, P.: Arteriography of the adrenals. Radiology, 92:999-1005, Apr. 1969.
7. Rossi, P., Young, I. S., and Panke, W. F.: Techniques, usefulness, and hazards of arteriography of pheochromocytoma. J.A.M.A., 205:547-553, Aug. 1968.

NOTES

Pelvic Arteriogram (Triple Contrast Bladder Study and Gynecologic)

TRAY — Seldinger arteriogram

CATHETER — #7 single curve 80 cm. Selective hypogastric "p" shaped catheter.

OPAQUE MEDIA — 76% meglumine diatrizoate

INJECTION — 15 cc/sec for 3 sec into distal aorta.
6 to 10 cc/sec for 3 sec into selective hypogastric

FILM RATE — 1 film per sec for 10 sec
Initial filming is A-P followed by suitable obliques

Perivesicle Air Equipment

Large Asepto syringe for filling bladder with air.
#17G spinal needle (perivesicle gas). Sterile rubber tubing for O_2 50 cc glass syringe and 3-way stopcock.

NOTES Triple Contrast

A #17 gauge spinal needle is introduced at a point 2 cm above and 2 cm lateral to the symphysis pubis bilaterally under local anesthesia and 500-600 cc of oxygen introduced into the perivesicle space. This is done *under fluoroscopic control.* A 50 ml glass syringe with a 3-way stopcock is used. The patient is kept in 30° Trendelenberg position to prevent the gas from rising.

Following instillation of the oxygen, a #7 single curve catheter is placed in the aorta via the percutaneous route with the tip just above the aortic bifurcation. A test dose of contrast is given and the position checked fluoroscopically. The bladder is then filled with air via a previously placed Foley catheter and the catheter clamped. Injection and filming are then carried out, (4).

Selective hypogastric. The hypogastric opposite the femoral entered can frequently be entered with a single or double curve catheter. A malleable "p" shaped catheter is convenient on the same side, (1, 9).

REFERENCES

1. Altemus, R.: Selective catheterization of the hypogastric arteries: Advantages and discussion of technic. Radiology, 91:484-487, Sept. 1968.
2. Benson, R. C., Dotter, C. T., and Straube, K. R.: Percutaneous transfemoral aortography in gynecology and obstetrics. Amer. J. Ob. Gyn., 85:772-791, Mar. 1963.
3. Brewis, R. A. L., and Bagshawe, K. D.: Pelvic arteriography in invasive trophoblastic neoplasia. Brit. J. Radiology, 41:481-495, July 1968.
4. Lacy, S. S., Whitley, J. E., and Cox, C. E.: Vesical arteriography: An adjunct to staging of bladder tumors. Brit J. Urology, 42: 50-55, 1970.
5. Lang, E. K.: Arteriography in gynecology. Radiol. Clin. of N. A., 5:133-149, Apr. 1967.
6. Lang, E. K., Nourse, M. H., Wishard, W. N., and Mertz, J. H. O.: The accuracy of preoperative staging of bladder tumors by arteriography: a 5-year study. J. Urol., 95:363-367, Mar. 1966.
7. Lang, E. K., Wishard, W. N., Nourse, M. H., and Mertz, J. H. O.: Retrograde arteriography in the diagnosis of bladder tumors. J. Urol., 89:422-426, Mar. 1963.
8. Nilsson, J.: Angiography in tumours of the urinary bladder. Acta Radiologica: Suppl. 263, 1967.
9. Meng, C. H., and Elkin, M.: Gynecologic angiography. Seminars in Roentgen., 4:267-279, July 1969.
10. Mikaelsson, C. G.: Polythene catheter of new shape for percutaneous selective catheterization. Acta Radiologica (Diag.), 3:581-591, Dec. 1965.

NOTES

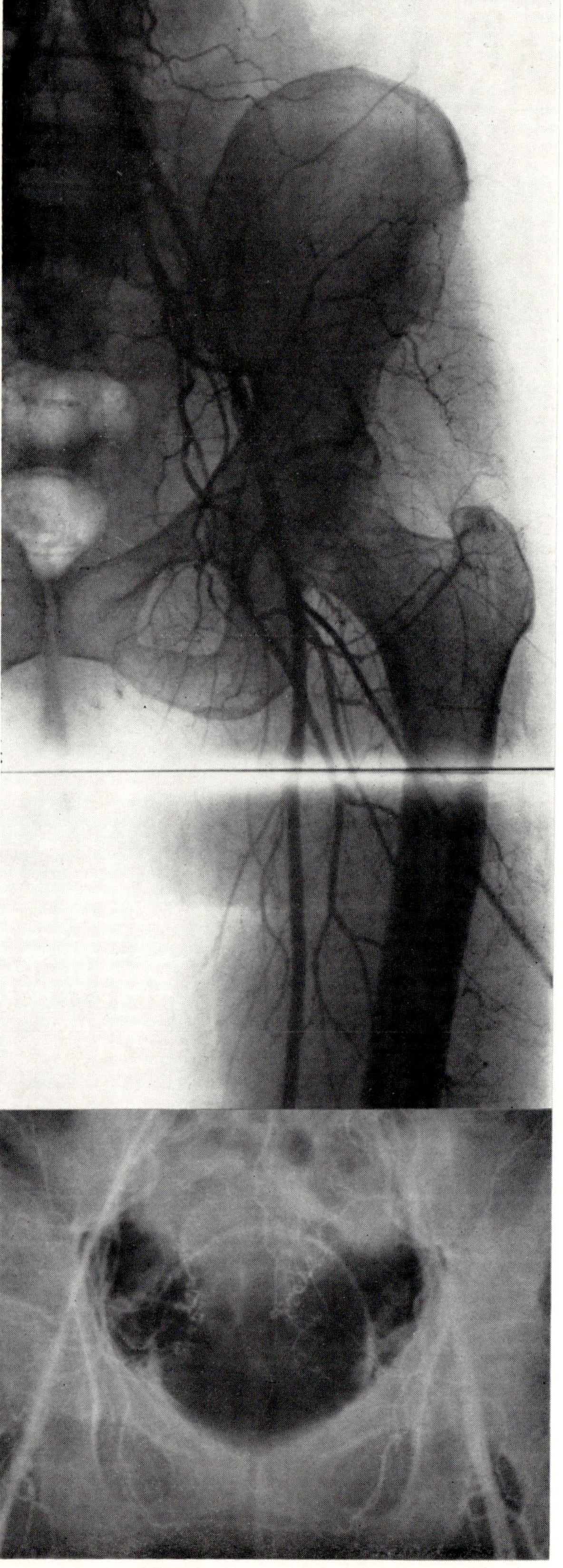

FIGURE 15. Pelvic Arteriogram.

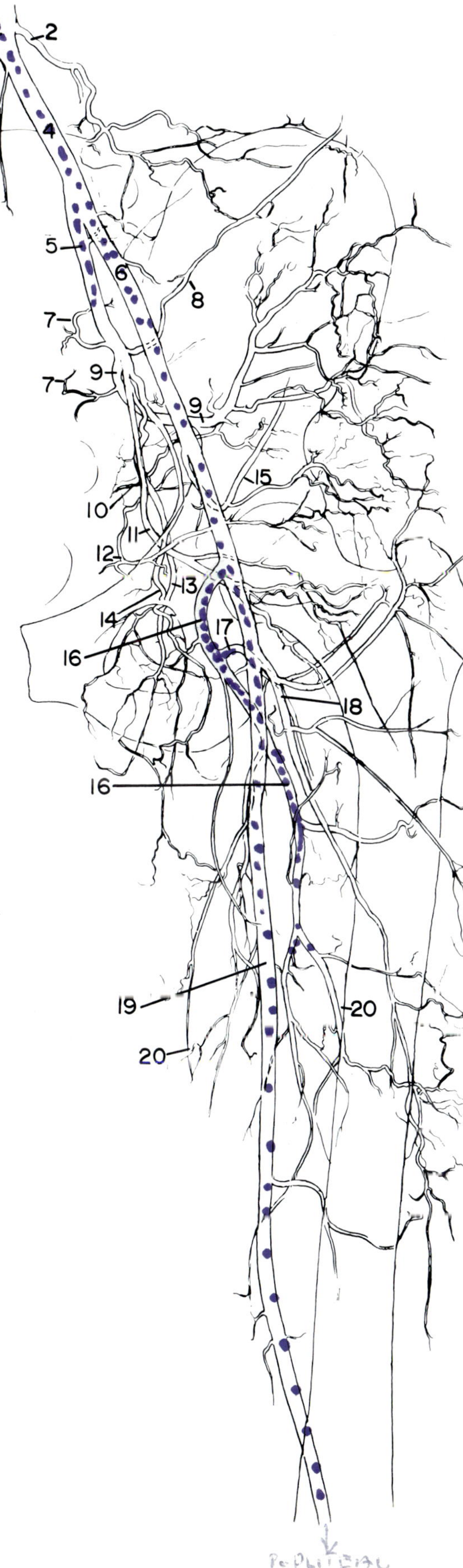

1. Abdominal aorta
2. Lumbar A.
3. Superior sacral A.
4. Common iliac A.
6. External iliac A.
5. Internal iliac A. (hypogastric)
7. Lateral sacral arteries (posterior division of internal iliac)
8. Iliolumbar A. (posterior division)
9. Superior gluteal A. (posterior division)
10. Vesicular arteries (anterior division internal iliac)
11. Inferior gluteal A. (anterior division)
12. External pudendal A. (from femoral A.)
13. Internal pudendal A. (anterior division)
14. Obturator A. (anterior division)
15. Deep circumflex iliac A.
16. Profunda femoris A. (deep femoral A.)
17. Medial circumflex femoral A.
18. Lateral circumflex femoral A.
19. Superficial femoral A.
20. Muscular branches (perforating branches)

Inferior Vena Cavogram

MATERIALS: 2 — 50 cc syringes
2 — #16 teflon sheath needles (2 ½ inch)
2 — packages venotubing
2 — bottles saline for slow infusion through needles
2 — J guide wire (30 cm)

OPAQUE MEDIA — 76% meglumine diathrizoate

INJECTION RATE — 30 cc each femoral vein by hand injection, catheter in low IVC — 20 cc/sec for 3 sec.

FILM RATE — 1/sec for 6 sec (biplane). Start filming with 10 cc left to inject.

NOTES:

Percutaneous insertion of needles bilaterally into femoral veins and pass guide wire to help thread teflon sheaths. Then attach to infusion until ready to inject. If both sides connot be injected, insert guide wire and place #8 single curve (80 cm) catheter in low inferior vena cava or in iliac vein and place a B.P. tourniquet around the opposite thigh to occlude venous return and prevent dilution of contrast media.

At the level of L-2 in the lateral view, there is usually indentation and anterior displacement of the vena cava as the right renal artery passes behind it to reach the right kidney. There are usually negative jets of unopacified blood entering the vena cava from the renal and hepatic veins. These may cause dilution or streaming of the contrast media. There is frequent normal thinning of the contrast media in the left iliac vein in the area of the fifth lumbar vertebra. This impression is caused by the right iliac artery crossing the vein. Visualization of the ascending lumbar veins, and sacral collaterals is not a definite sign of abnormality so long as the definitive channel is opacified.

REFERENCES

1. Blazek, J. V., Clark, R. L., and Herron, C. S.: Cavography following plication of the inferior vena cava. Amer. J. Roentgenol., 98:888-897, Dec. 1966.
2. Ferris, E. J., Vittimberga, F. J., Byrne, J. J., Nabseth, D. C., and Shapiro, J. H.: The inferior vena cava after ligation and plication; a study of collateral routes. Radiology, 89:1-10, July, 1967.
3. Fletcher, E. W. L., and Thomas, M. L.: Chronic post-thrombotic obstruction of inferior vena cava investigated by cavography; a report of 11 cases. Amer. J. Roentgenol., 102:363-371, Feb. 1968.
4. Hillman, D. C., and Tristan, T. A.: Inferior vena cavography in the detection of abdominal extension of pelvic cancer. Radiology, 81:416-427, Sept. 1963.
5. Holtz, S., and Powers, W. E.: Inferior vena cavagrams. Radiology, 78:583-590, Apr. 1960.
6. Kerr, M. G., Scott, D. B., and Samuel, E.: Studies of the inferior vena cava in late pregnancy. Brit. Med. J., 1:532-533, Feb. 1964.

NOTES

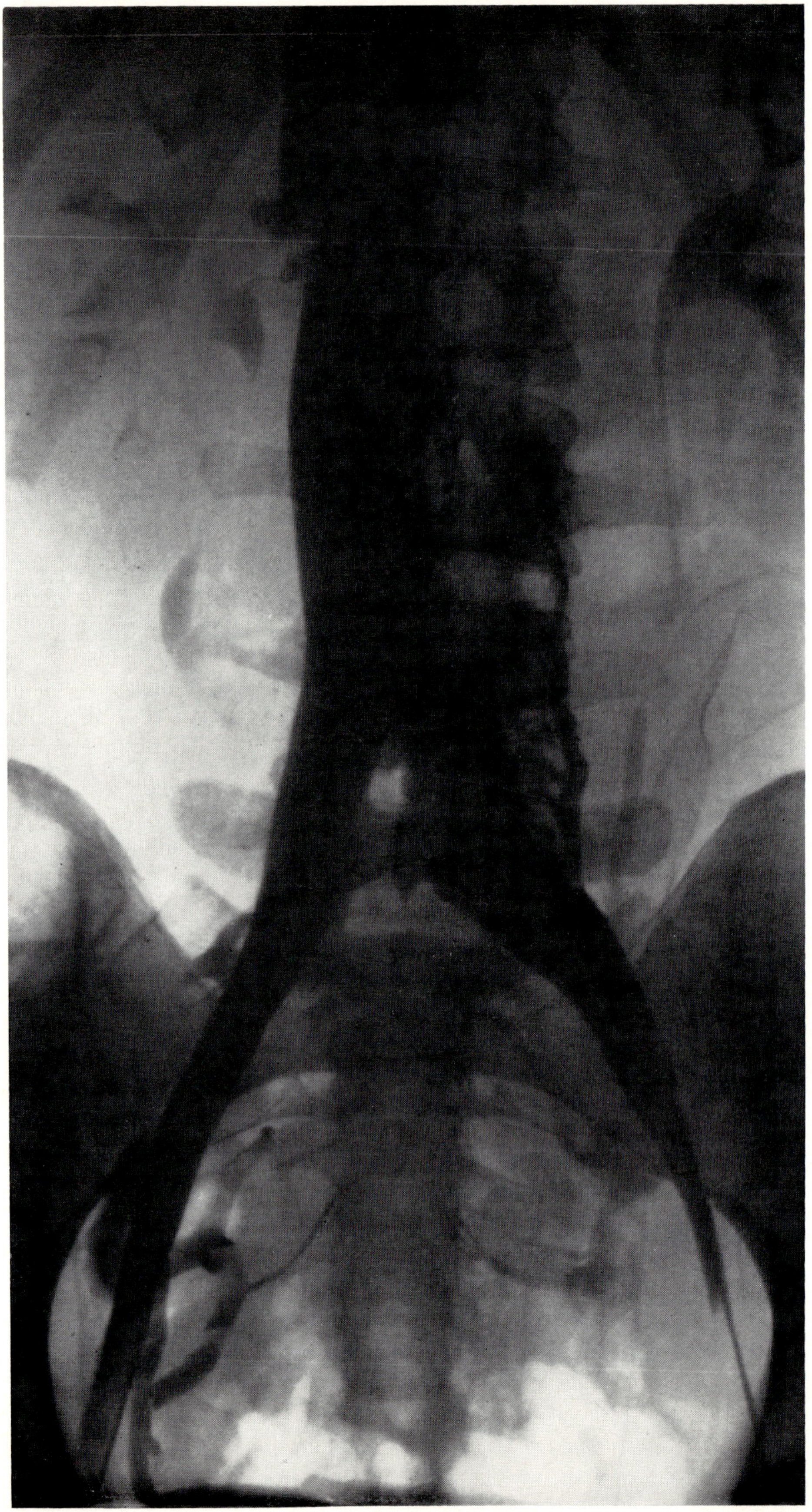

FIGURE 16. Inferior Vena Cavogram.

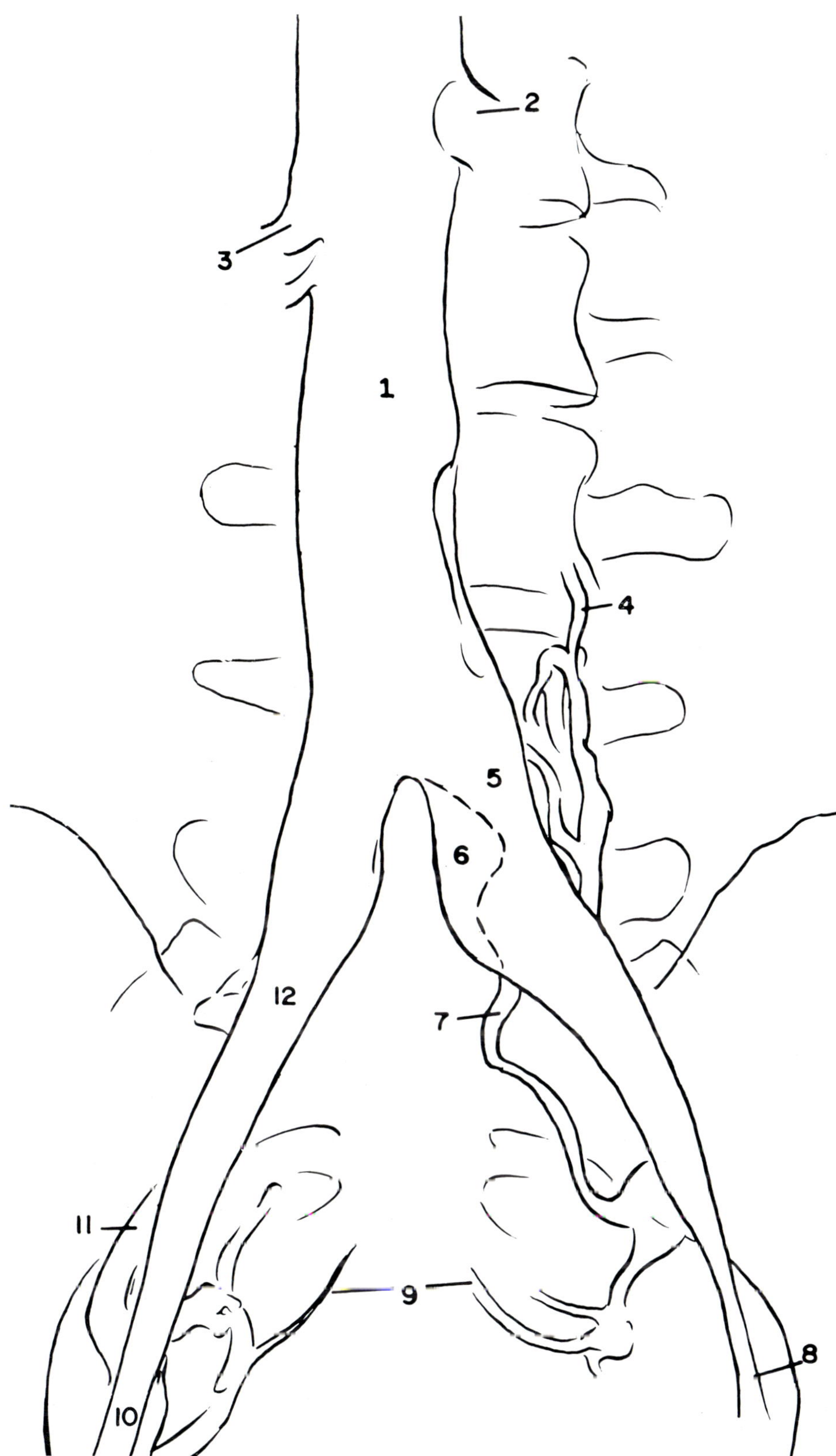

1. Inferior vena cava
2. Left renal vein refluxed with dilution
3. Right renal vein refluxed with dilution
4. Ascending lumbar vein (this is not an abnormal finding on left)
5. Left common iliac vein
6. Normal area of lucency caused by compression of vein by right iliac A.
7. Median sacral vein
8. "Jet" effect from injection
9. Lateral sacral vein
10. External iliac vein
11. Internal iliac vein
12. Right common iliac vein

PERIPHERAL

Brachial Arteriogram

TRAY — Seldinger arteriogram or angiogram tray
CATHETER — #7 single curve or headhunter catheter
OPAQUE MEDIA — 60% meglumine diatrizoate or iothalamate
INJECTION RATE — 8-10 cc/sec for 2-3 sec
NOTES

Technique if studying inlet syndrome, do both arms with arms neutral and above head.

Arterial puncture of brachial is performed as previously described for cerebral retrograde brachial with filming over hand, forearm or upper arm.

REFERENCES

1. Haimovici, H., and Caplan, L. H.: Arterial thrombosis complicating thoracic outlet syndrome; arteriographic considerations. Radiology, 87:462-464, Sept. 1966.
2. Wellauer, J.: Arteriography. In. *Roentgen Diagnosis.* Volume I: *General Principles and Methods.* Edited by H. R. Schinz and others. 2nd American edition, New York, Grune & Stratton, 1968, ch. 15, pp. 279-301.

NOTES

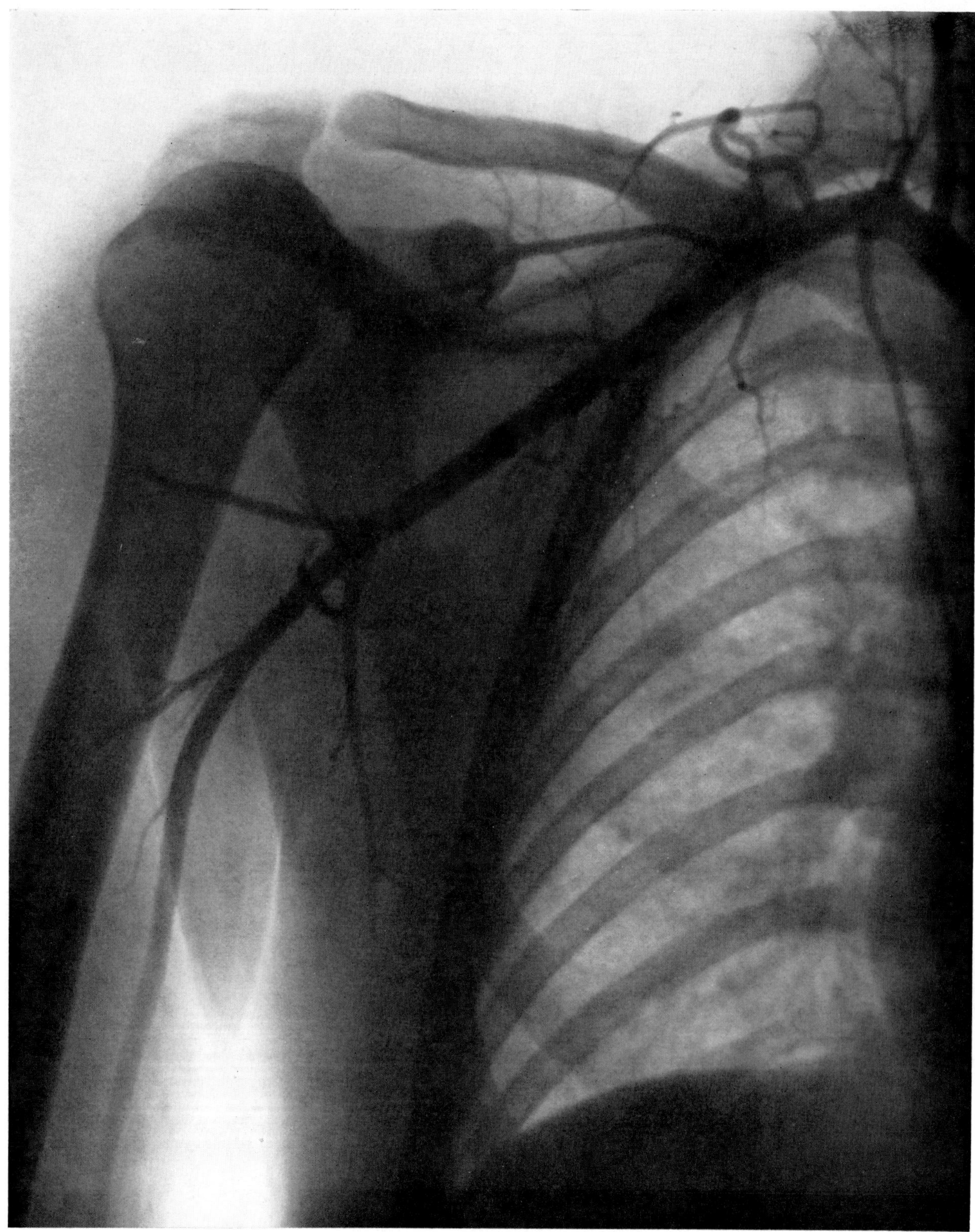

FIGURE 17. Brachial Arteriogram.

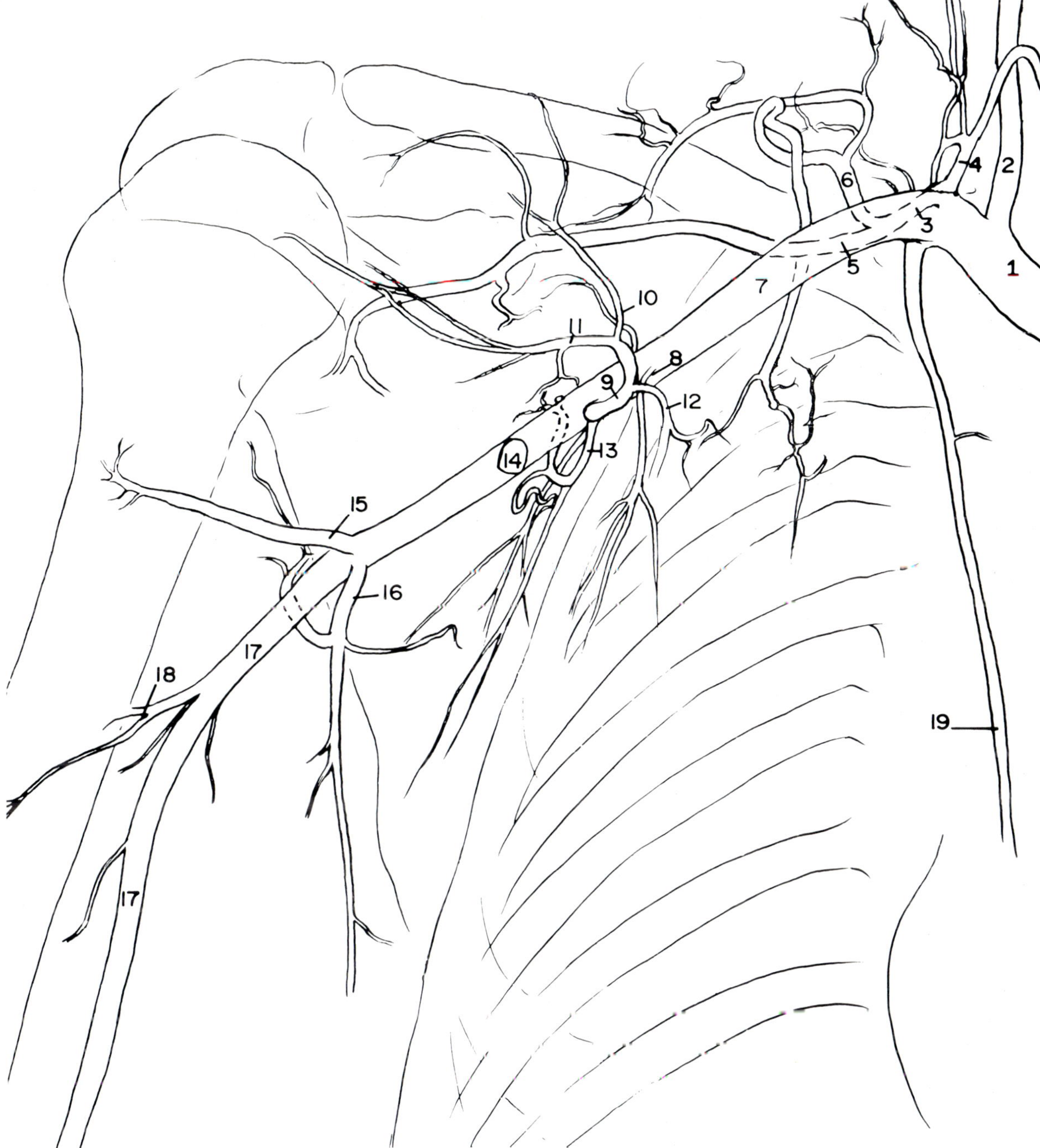

1. Subclavian A.
2. Vertebral A.
3. Thyrocervical trunk
4. Inferior thyroid A. (from thyrocervical trunk)
5. Suprascapular A. (from thyrocervical trunk)
6. Transverse cervical A.
7. Axillary A.
8. Highest thoracic A.
9. Thoraco-acromial trunk
10. Acromial branch of thoraco-acromial
11. Deltoid branch of thoraco-acromial
12. Pectoral branch of thoraco-acromial
13. Lateral thoracic A.
14. Metallic object soft tissues
15. Circumflex humeral A.
16. Subscapular A.
17. Brachial A.
18. Deep brachial A.
19. Internal mammary A.

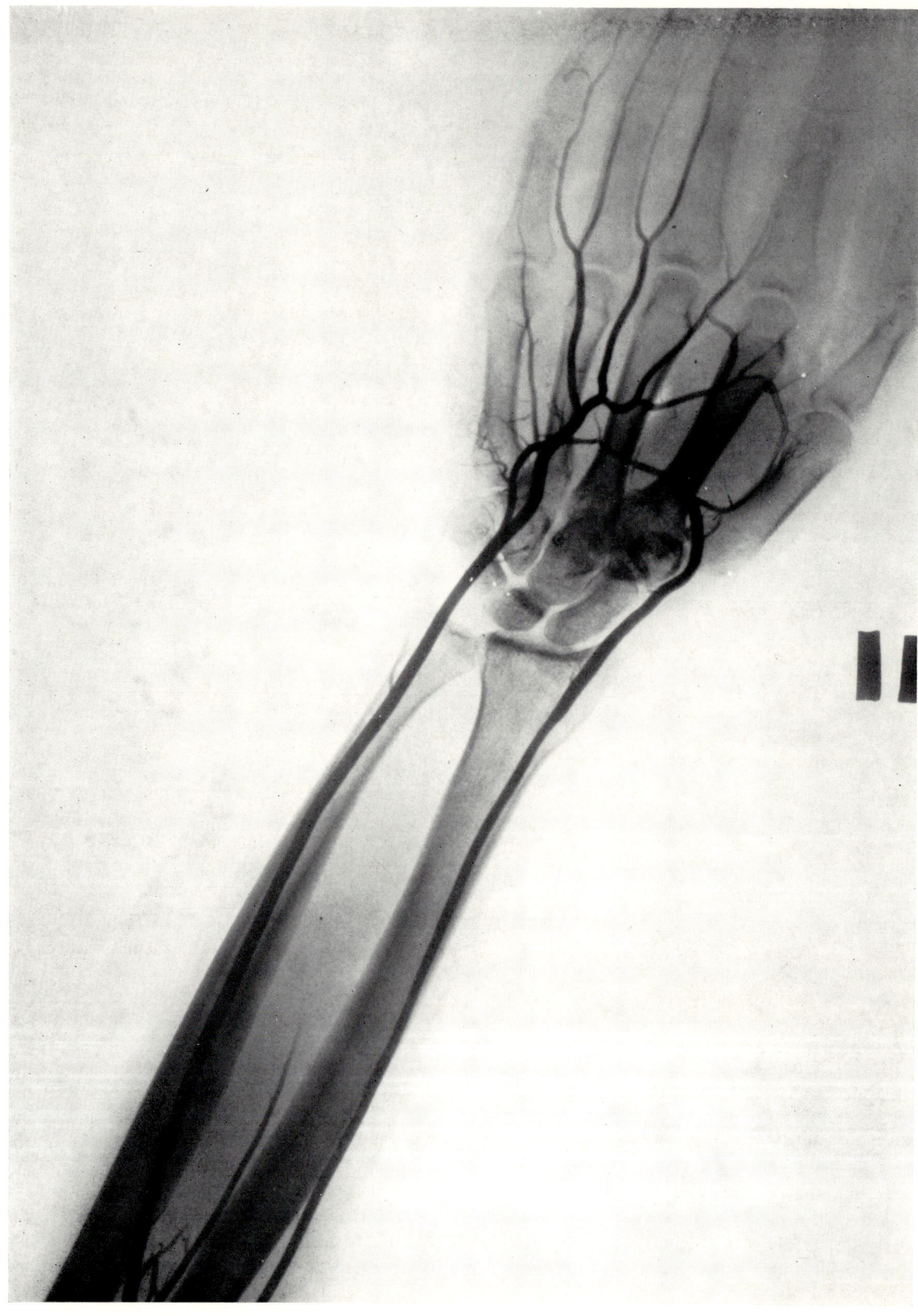

FIGURE 18. Forearm Arteriogram.

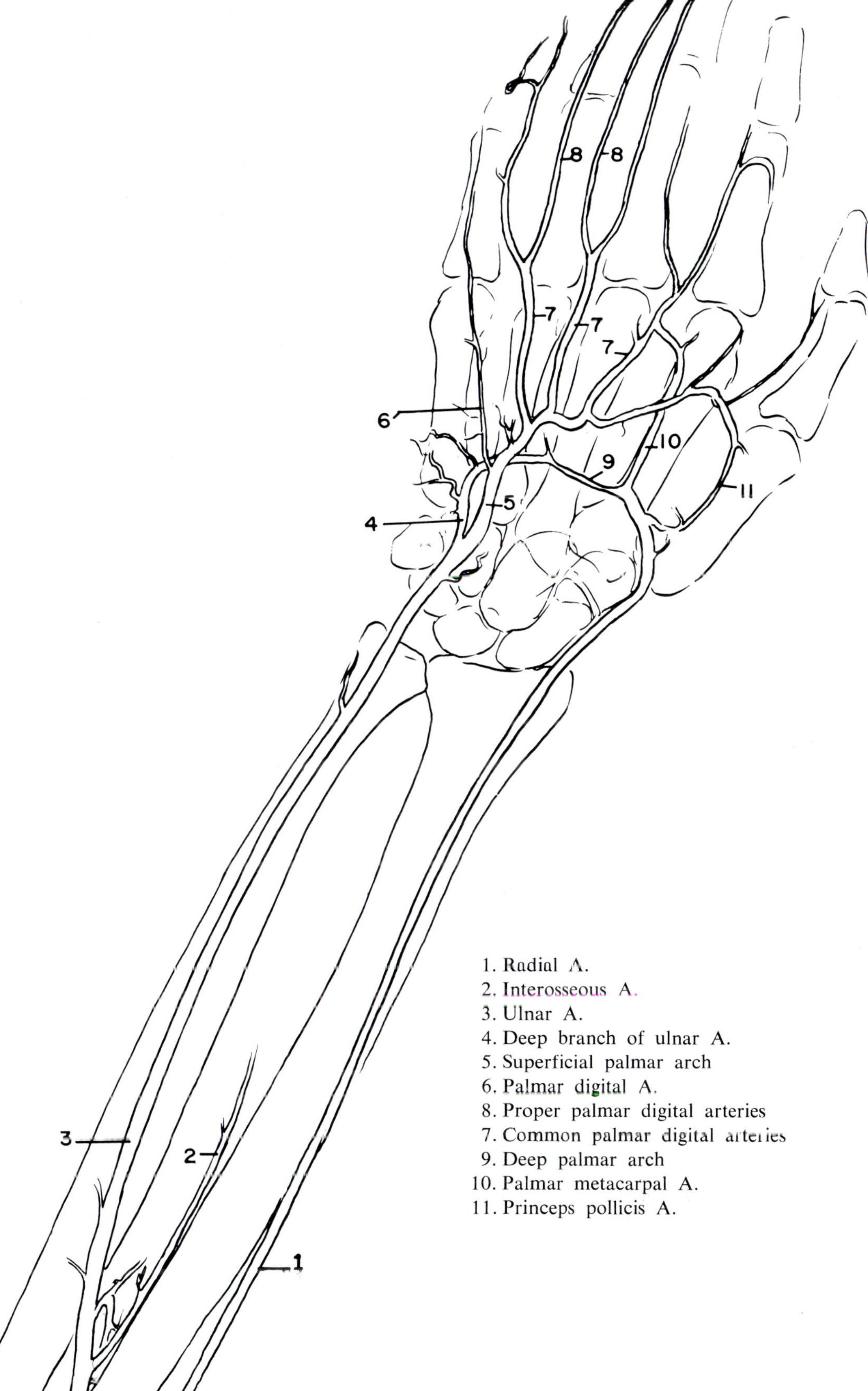

1. Radial A.
2. Interosseous A.
3. Ulnar A.
4. Deep branch of ulnar A.
5. Superficial palmar arch
6. Palmar digital A.
8. Proper palmar digital arteries
7. Common palmar digital arteries
9. Deep palmar arch
10. Palmar metacarpal A.
11. Princeps pollicis A.

Femoral Arteriogram

TRAY — Seldinger arteriogram
CATHETER OR NEEDLE — #7 straight or single curve (80 cm)
#16 teflon sheath needle (direct puncture 2 ½ inch
#18 arterial (direct puncture)
OPAQUE MEDIA — 76% meglumine diatriozoate
INJECTION RATE — Into distal aorta 10-15 cc/sec for 3-4 sec
Direct puncture per femoral 8-10 cc/sec for 2-3 sec.
FILM RATE — 0 sec (near end of injection)
2 sec
4 sec
6 sec
10 sec
14 sec
OR with obvious necrotic changes in feet
0 sec
3 sec
6 sec
9 sec
13 sec
17 sec

NOTES

Since most people with occlusive disease have difficulties bilaterally, placement of a catheter in the distal aorta is the technique of choice, preferably by way of the percutaneous femoral route, but if this is not possible, by translumbar or percutaneous axillary puncture. The catheter is placed just about the aortic bifurcation (about L-3), and a test injection is performed under flurosocopic control both for placement of the catheter and for sensitivity to the contrast medium. With either of the above filming sequences, the entire arterial tree of the pelvis and lower extremities is usually visualized with one injection.

If direct arterial puncture is performed, a teflon sheath is threaded into the arterial lumen maintaining a good pulsatile flow of blood. If an injector is used, 10 cc/sec for 2.5 sec usually is suficient to reflux the distal aorta (according to run-off). If the injection is manually, a larger amount is usually necessary to develop the flow-pressure relationship to reflux the distal aorta and exclude obstruction of the proximal iliac. The teflon sheath is attached to venotubing which has a clamp which can be closed at the end of injection. The tubing and clamp allow the operator to remove himself from the primary radiation beam. Filming is started with 10 cc of contrast medium left to inject.

REFERENCES

1. Cockshott, W. P., Evans, K. T.: The place of soft tissue arteriography. Brit. J. Radiology, 37:367-375, May 1964.
2. Dotter, C. T., Rosch, J., and Judkins, M. P.: Transluminal dilatation of atherosclerotic stenosis. Surg., Gynec. Obstet., 127:794-804, Oct. 1968.
3. Fridenberg, M. J., and Perez, C. A.: Collateral circulation in aorto-iliofemoral occlusive disease; as demonstrated by a unilateral percutaneous common femoral artery needle injection. Amer. J. Roentgenol., 94:145-158, May 1965.
4. Haimovici, H., Shapiro, J. H., and Jacobson, H. G.: Serial femoral arteriography in occlusive disease; clinical-roentgenologic considerations with a new classification of occlusive patterns. Amer. J. Roentgenol., 83:1042-1062, June 1960.
5. Halpern, M., and Freiberger, R. H.: Arteriography in orthopedics. Amer. J. Roentgenol., 94:194-206, May 1965.
6. Kahn, P. C., and Callow, A. D.: Selective vasodilatation as an aid to angiography. Amer. J. Roentgenol., 94:213-220. May 1965.
7. Lagergren, C., Lindbom, A., and Söderberg, G.: Vascularization of fibromatous and fibrosarcomatous tumors; histopathologic, microangiographic, and angiographic studies. Acta Radiologica, 53:1-16, Jan. 1960.
8. Sammons, B. P., and Mahin, H. P.: New technique of contrast visualization of the distal aorta, pelvic and lower extremity arterial system in obliterative vascular disease. Amer. J. Roentgenol., 81:835-840, May 1959.
9. Skinner, G. B.: The use of cinefluorography in peripheral arteriography. Amer. J. Roentgenol., 95:745-750, Nov. 1965.

NOTES

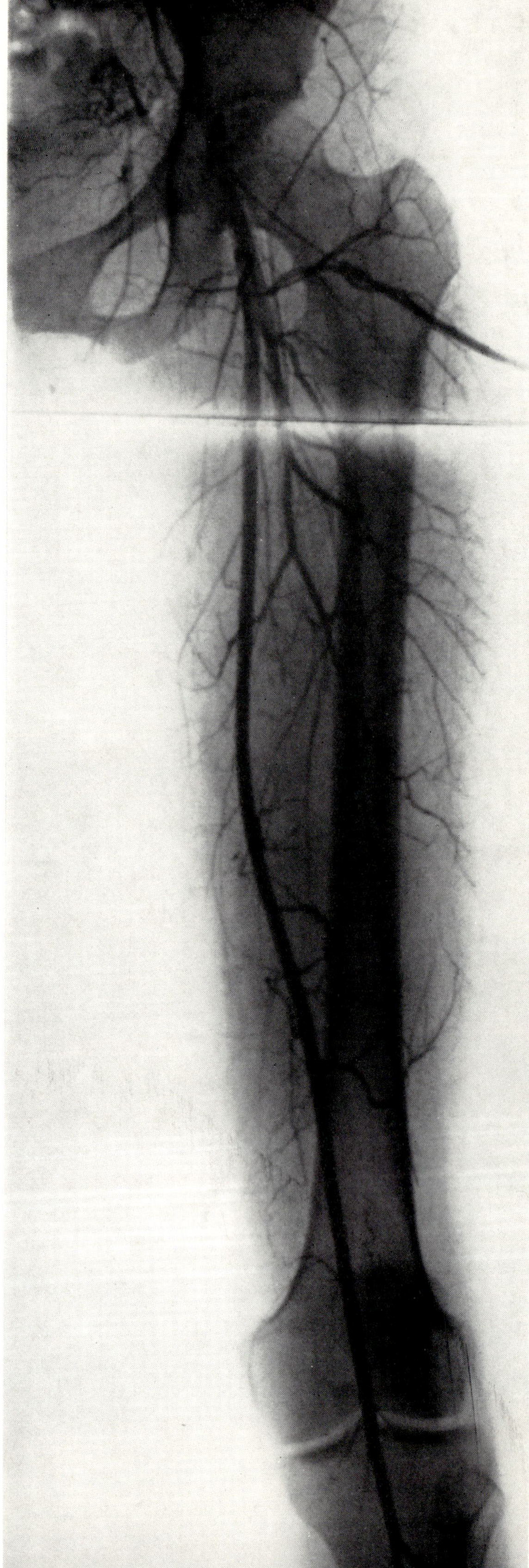

FIGURE 19. Femoral Arteriogram (thigh).

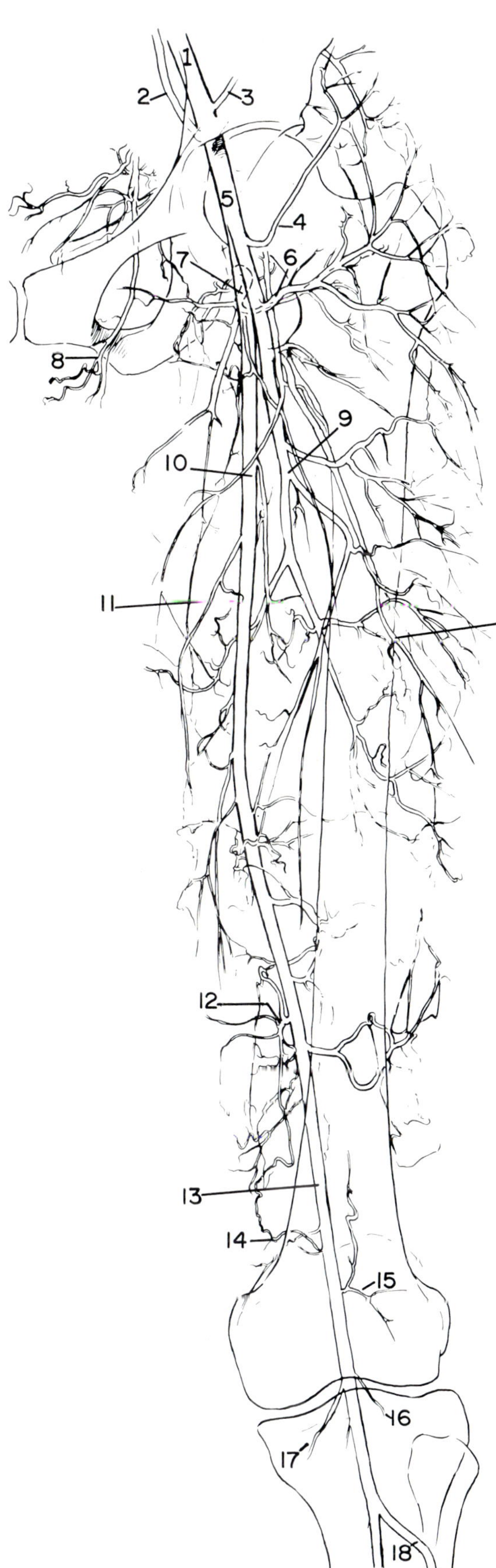

1. External iliac A.
2. Inferior epigastric
3. Deep circumflex iliac A.
4. Superficial circumflex iliac A.
5. Femoral A.
6. Lateral circumflex femoral
7. Medial circumflex femoral
8. Internal pudendal A.
9. Profunda femoris A. (Deep femoral A.)
10. Superficial femoris (Superficial femoral A.)
11. Muscular arteries (perforating arteries)
12. Descending genicular A.
13. Popliteal A.
14. Medial superior genicular A.
15. Lateral superior genicular A.
16. Lateral inferior genicular A.
17. Medial inferior genicular A.
18. Anterior tibial A.

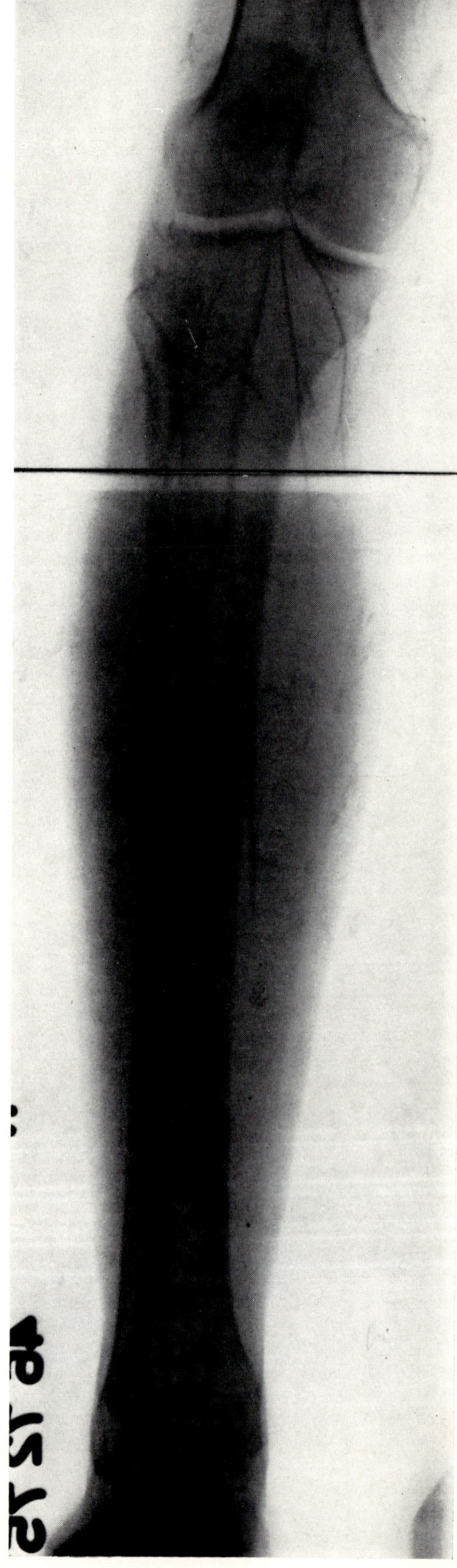

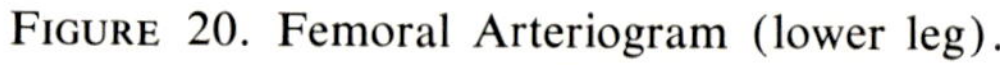

Figure 20. Femoral Arteriogram (lower leg).

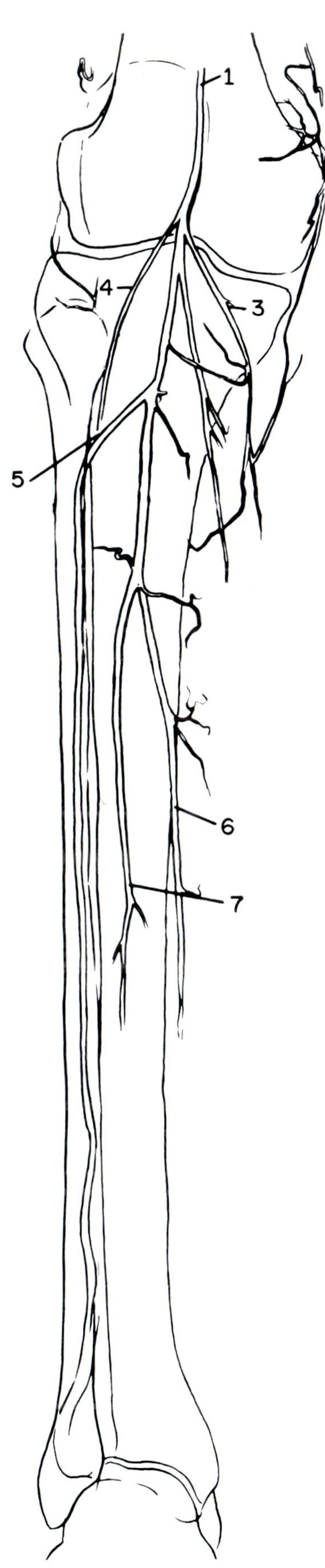

1. Popliteal A.
2. Saphenous branch of descending genicular A.
3. Inferior medial genicular A.
4. Inferior lateral genicular A.
5. Anterior tibial A.
6. Posterior tibial A.
7. Peroneal A. (Fibular A.)

Venograms, Lower Extremity

EQUIPMENT — 2 #19 scalp vein needles
(2) 50 cc syringes
2 Venotubes
2 bottles of dextrose and water or one bottle and Y set-up.

OPAQUE MEDIA — 50 cc 30% meglumine diatrizoate or iothalamate. Hand injected bilaterally into the vein of dorsum of foot.

TOURNIQUETS — Place above ankle to visualize deep veins of the calf.

FILM RATE — Films at:
0 sec (10 cc left to inject)
20 sec
40 sec
60 sec
90 sec
110 sec

With 20 sec between films, the legs may be placed in a lateral projection for at least one film. This should be practiced with patient prior to study.

INFUSION — 50 cc of Renografin plus 50 cc of D_5 H_20 in I-V set-up, into dorsum of each foot through a #19 scalp vein needle. Near the end of the infusion take two films 30 sec apart. I-V set-up of D_5 H_20 for infusion while films are being reviewed and to prevent chemical reaction in veins used during *both* procedures.

NOTES

Keep knees slightly flexed in AP shots or film in lateral, to prevent fascial artefact at knee. A cotton roll under the knee will also produce an artefact.

Infusion venograms are valuable for visualization of the entire venous system of the legs and pelvis and is particuarly helpful in defining thrombotic disease. It will not determine competence of perforators and both studies are usually done in the work-up of patients with varicose veins. Only the infusion technique is performed in thrombotic problems.

Tourniquets above the knees may be of help in visualizing the deep pelvic veins on the routine study.

REFERENCES

1. Almen, T., and Nylander, G.: False signs of thrombosis in lower leg phlebography. Acta Radiologica (Diag.), 2:345-352, July 1964.
2. Baltaxe, H. A., Meade, J. W., Temes, G. D., Saunders, J., and Mueller, C. B.: Lymphatic and venous examination of the postphlebitic extremity. Radiology, 91:478-483, Sept. 1968.
3. Borgström, S., Greitz, T., Van der Linden, W., Molin, J., and Rudics, I.: Ascending phlebography in fresh thrombosis of the lower limb. Amer. J. Roentgenol., 94:207-212, May, 1965.
4. DeWeese, J. A., and Rogoff, S.: Functional ascending phlebography of the lower extremity by serial long film technique. Amer. J. Roentgenol., 81:841-854, May 1959.
5. Greitz, T.: Ascending phlebography in venous insufficiency. Acta Radiologica, 44:145-162, Aug. 1955.
6. Gretiz, T.: Phlebography of the normal leg. Acta Radiologica, 44:1-20, July 1955.
7. Nylander, G.: Lower leg phlebography by an improved technique. Acta Radiologica, 57:348-352, Sept. 1962.
8. Wegner, G. P., Flaherty, T. T., and Crummy, A. B.: Intraosseous lower extremity venography. Arch. Surg., 98:105-110, Jan. 1969.

NOTES

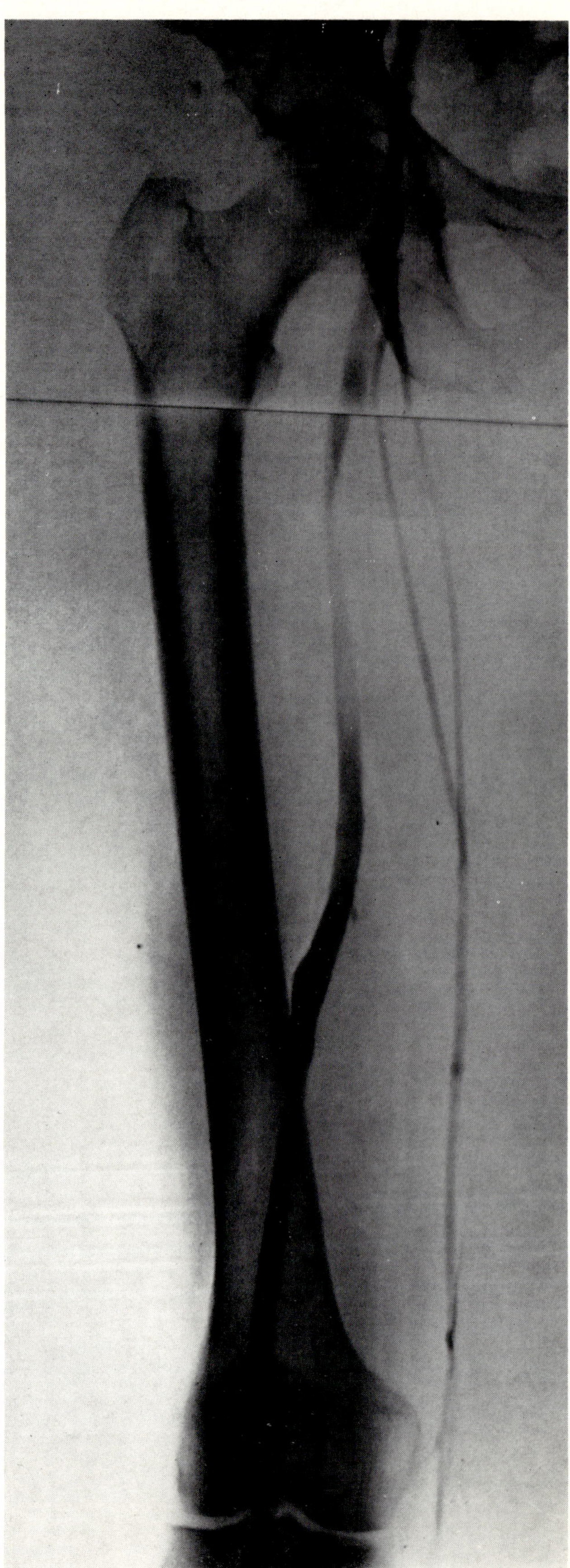

FIGURE 21. Venograms (thigh).

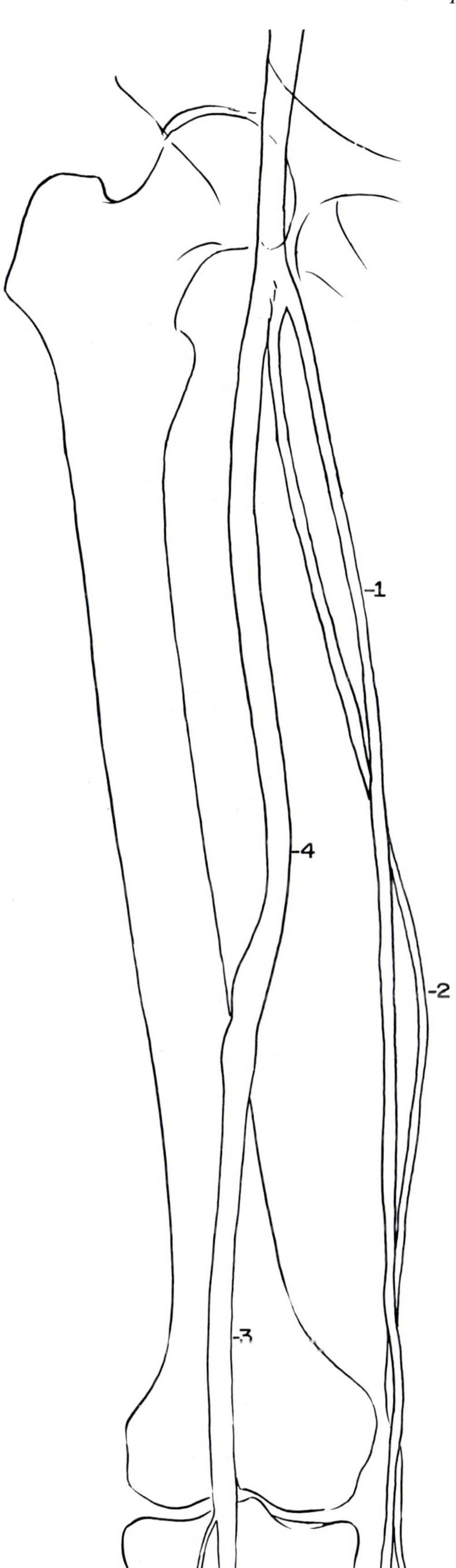

1. Greater saphenous V.
2. Accessory greater saphenous V.
3. Popliteal V.
4. Deep femoral V.

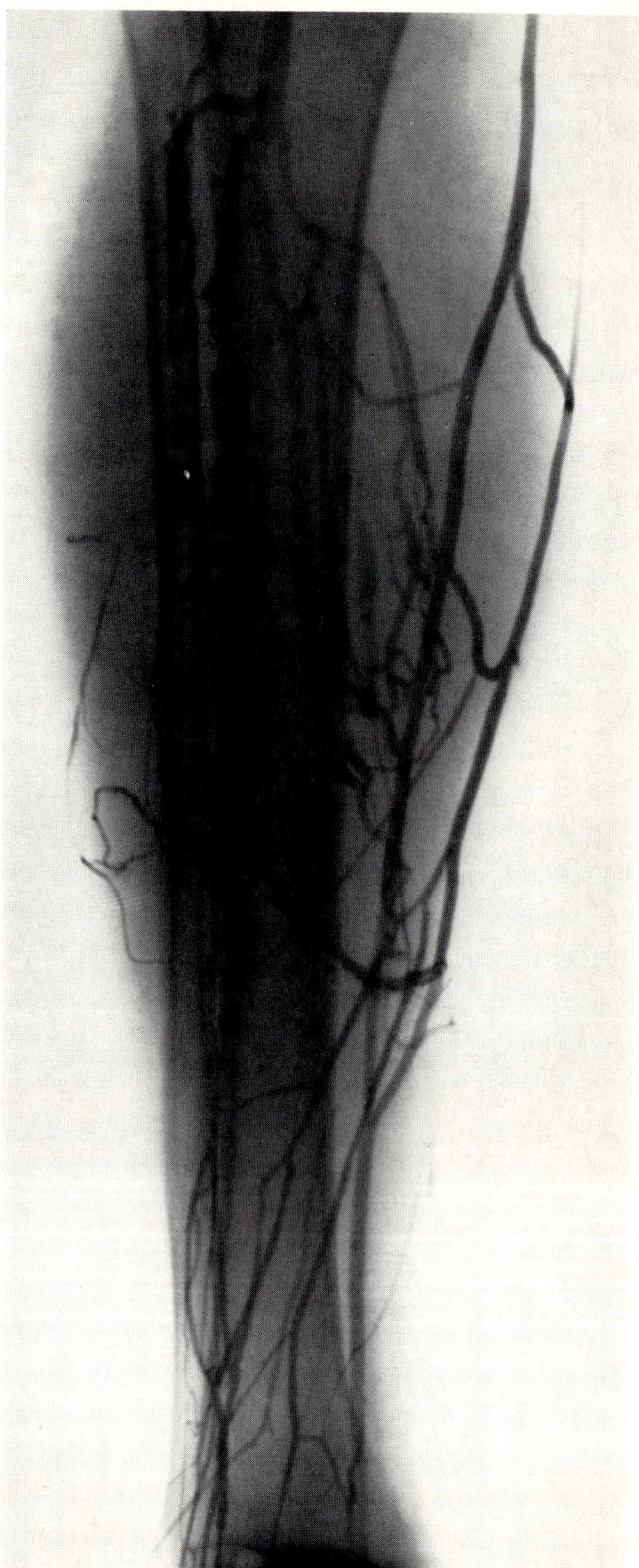

FIGURE 22. Venogram (lower leg).

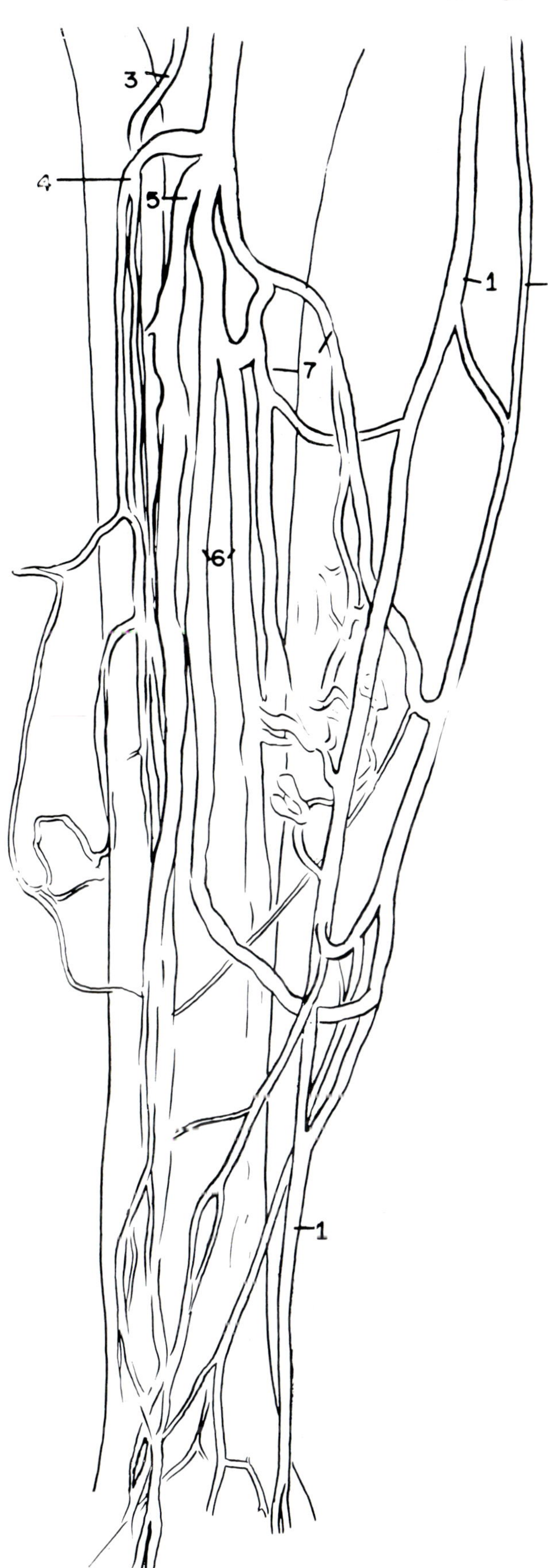

1. Greater saphenous V.
2. Accessory greater saphenous V.
3. Lesser saphenous V.
4. Ant. tibial veins
5. Peroneal V.
6. Posterior tibial veins
7. Calf (sural) veins

References To Additional Techniques And Procedures

GENERAL AND PEDIATRIC

1. Ahlberg, N. E., Bartley, O., and Chidekel, N.: Venous arteriography; a modified technique and indications for its use. Acta. Radiologica (Diag.), 7:321-330, July 1968.
2. Amplatz, K., and Harner, R.: A new subclavian artery catheterization technic; Preliminary report. Radiology, 78:963-966, June 1962.
3. Boijsen, E.: Selective visceral angiography using a percutaneous axillary technique. Brit. J. Radiology, 39:414-421, June 1966.
4. Bron, K. M., Riley, R. R., and Girdany, B. R.: Pediatric arteriography in abdominal and extremity lesions; clinical experience, indications, and technic. Radiology, 92:1241-1255, May 1969.
5. Kaplan, L. S., Helff, J. R., and Kirchner, R. G.: The application of a pressurized infusor to arteriography. Radiology, 84:330-332, Feb. 1965.
6. Kessler, R. E., and Zimmon, D. S.: Umbilical vein angiography. Radiology, 87:841-844, Nov. 1966.
7. Nebesar, R. A., Fleischli, D. J., Pollard, J. J., and Griscom, N. T.: Arteriography in infants and children; with emphasis on the Seldinger technique and abdominal diseases. Amer. J. Roentgenol., 106:81-91, May 1969.
8. Peck, D. R., Lowman, R. M.: Roentgen aspects of umbilical vascular catheterization in the newborn: the problem of catheter placement. Radiology, 89:874-877, Nov. 1967.
9. Poser, C. M., and Taveras, J. M.: Clinical aspects of cerebral angiography in children. Pediatrics, 16:73-80, July 1955.
10. Viamonte, M., and Stevens, R. C.: Guided angiography. Amer. J. Roentgenol., 94:30-39, May 1965.

CENTRAL NERVOUS SYSTEM

1. DiChiro, G., Doppman, J., and Ommaya, A. K.: Selective arteriography of arteriovenous aneurysms of spinal cord. Radiology, 88:1065-1077, June 1967.
2. Loyd, G. A. S.: A technique for arteriography of the orbit. Brit. J. Radiology, 42:252-255, April 1969.
3. McNulty, J. G.: Phlebography of the orbital venous system and the cavernous sinus. Brit. J. Radiology, 42:113-121, Feb. 1969.
4. Wilson, G. H., and Hanafee, W. N.: Angiographic findings in 16 patients with juvenile nasopharyngeal angiofibroma. Radiology, 92:279-284, Feb. 1969.

THORACIC

1. Boijsen, E., and Reuter, S. R.: Subclavian and internal mammary angiography in the evaluation of the anterior mediastinal masses. Amer. Roentgenol., 98:447-450, Oct. 1966.
2. Doppman, J. L., Hammond, W. G., Nelson, G. L., Evans, R. G., and Ketchan, A. S.: Staining of parathyroid adenomas by selective arteriography. Radiology, 92:527-530, Mar. 1969.
3. Feldman, F., Habif, D. V., Fleming, R. J., Kanter, I. E., Seaman, W. B.: Arteriography of the breast. Radiology, 89:1053-1061, Dec. 1967.
4. Judkins, M. P.: Percutaneous transfemoral selective coronary arteriography. Radiol. Clin. of N. A., 6:467-492, Dec. 1968.
5. Newton, T. H., and Eisenberg, E.: Angiography of parathyroid adenomas. Radiology, 86:843-850, May 1966.
6. Nordenström, B.: A method of angiography of azygos vein and the anterior internal venous plexus of the spine. Acta Radiologica, 44:201-208, Sept. 1965.
7. Seldinger, S. I.: Localization of parathyroid adenomata by arteriography. Acta Radiologica, 42: 353-366, Nov. 1954.
8. Takahashi, M., Ishibashi, T., and Kawanami, H.: Angiographic diagnosis of benign and malignant tumors of the thyroid. Radiology, 92:520-526, Mar. 1969.
9. Viamonte, M., Parks, R. E., and Smoak, W. M.: Guided catheterization of the bronchial arteries. Radiology, 85:205-230, Aug. 1965.
10. Wickbom, I., Zachrisson, B. F., and Heimann, P.: Thyroid angiography. Acta Radiologica (Diag.), 6:497-512, Nov 1967.

ABDOMINAL

1. Ahlberg, N. E., Bartley, O., Chidekel, N., and Fritjofsson, A.: Phlebography in varicocele scroti. Acta Radiologica (Diag.) 4:517-528, Sept. 1966.
2. Chidekel, N.: Female pelvic veins demonstrated by selective renal phlebography with particular reference to pelvic varicosities. Acta Radiologica (Diag.), 7:193-211, May 1968.
3. Chidekel, N., and Edlundh, K. O.: Transuterine phlebography with particular reference to pelvic varicosities. Acta Radiologica (Diag.), 7:1-12, Jan. 1968.
4. Frates, R. E.: Selective angiography of the ovarian artery. Radiology, 92:1014-1019, April. 1969.
5. Jacobs, J B.: Selective gonadal venography. Radiology, 92:885-888, Mar. 1969.
6. Kahn, P. C., and Frates, R. E.: The value of angiography of the small branches of the abdominal aorta. Amer. J. Roentgenol., 102:407-417, Feb. 1968.
7. Lang, E. K., and Greer, J. L.: The value of pelvic arteriography for the staging of carcinoma of the cervix. Radiology, 92:1027-1034, Apr. 1969.
8. Mikaelsson, C. G.: Epinephro-phlebography in two cases of Conn's syndrome. Acta Radiologica (Diag.), 7:410-416, Sept. 1968.
9. Rösch, J., Grollman, J. H., and Steckel, R. J.: Arteriography in the diagnosis of gallbladder disease. Radiology, 92:1485-1491, June 1969.
10. Ruzicka, F. F., and Rossi, P.: Arterial portography; patterns of venous flow. Radiology, 92-777-787, Mar. 1969.

PERIPHERAL

1. Dotter, C. T., and Judkins, M. P.: Percutaneous transluminal treatment of arteriosclerotic obstruction. Radiology, 84:631-643, Apr. 1965.
2. Wegner, G. P., Flaherty, T. T., and Crummy, A. B.: Intraosseous lower extremity venography. Arch. Surg., 98:105-110, Jan. 1969.
3. Willerson, J. T., Thompson, R. H., Hookman, P., Herdt, J., and Decker, J. L.: Reserpine in Raynaud's disease and phenomenon; short-term response to intra-arterial injection. Ann. Int. Med., 72:17-27, Jan. 1970.

CURRENT REFERENCE BOOKS

1. Abrams, Herbert L.: *Angiography*. Boston, Little, Brown, 1961.
2. Beranbaum, Samuel L., and Meyers, Phillip H., eds.: *Special Procedures in Roentgen Diagnosis.* Springfield, Ill., Thomas, 1964.
3. Bierman, Howard R.: *Selective Arterial Catheterization. Diagnostic, Therapeutic and Investigative.* Springfield, Ill., Thomas, 1969.
4. Epstein, Bernard S.: *Pneumoencephalography and Cerebral Angiography*. Chicago, Year Book Medical Publishers, 1966.
5. Kincaid, Owings, W., ed.: *Renal Angiography*. Chicago, Year Book Medical Publishers, 1966.
6. Meschan, Isadore: *An Atlas of Normal Radiographic Anatomy,* 2nd ed. Philadelphia, Saunders, 1959.
7. Michels, Nicholas A.: *Blood Supply and Anatomy of the Upper Abdominal Organs.* Philadelphia, Lippincott, 1955.
8. Nebesar, Robert A., and others: *Celiac and Superior Mesenteric Arteries: Correlation of Angiograms and Dissections.* Boston, Little, Brown, 1969.
9. Schinz, Hans R., and others: *Roentgen Diagnosis. Volume 1: General Principles and Methods.* 2d American edition. New York, Grune & Stratton, 1968.
10. Schobinger, Robert A., and Ruzicka, Francis F., eds.: *Vascular Roentgenology; Arteriography, Phlebography, Lymphography*. New York, Macmillan, 1964.
11. Taveras, Juan M., and Wood, Ernest H.: *Diagnostic Neuroradiology*. Baltimore, Williams & Wilkins. 1964.
12. Toole, James F., ed.: *Special Techniques for Neurologic Diagnosis.* Contemporary Neurology Series, vol. 3. Philadelphia, Davis, 1969.
13. Viamonte, Manuel, and Parks, Raymond E., comp. and eds.: *Progress in Angiography*. Springfield, Ill., Thomas, 1964.
14. Wilson, McClure: *The Anatomical Foundation of Neuroradiology of the Brain.* Boston, Little, Brown, 1963.
15. Zhebök, Zoltan D.: *Technic of Roentgenologic Investigations.* Budapest, Akadémiai Kiadó, 1969.

Appendix

SUGGESTED TRAY CONTENTS*

Seldinger Tray

2 Medicine glasses for antiseptic
1 Sponge forceps
3 Steel basins (large, medium and small)
1 #11 surgical blade
4 Sterile towels
4 Towel clips
2 Curved hemostat, (one mosquito)
1 Stopcock
12 Sponges, 4″ x 4″
1 10 cc syringe
3 20 cc syringes
1 Teflon dilator

Cut-down Tray

2 Medicine glasses
1 Sponge forceps
3 Steel basins (large, medium, and small)
1 #15 surgical blade and handle
4 Sterile towels
4 Towel clips
1 Small self retaining retractor (mastoid-type)
2 Vein retractors
4 Curved hemostats (mosquito)
2 Straight hemostats (mosquito)
1 Stopcock
2 Vessel tapes (fabric or rubber)
12 Sponges, 4″ x 4″
3 10 cc syringes
3 20 cc syringes
1 Fine opthalmologic forceps
1 Fine opthalmologic scissors
1 Small pair of scissors
1 Thumb forceps without teeth
2 Curved cutting needles (medium)
3-0 silk
1 Needleholder (small)

*Disposable 25 and 21 gauge needles, arteriographic needles, venotube and high pressure connectors, guide wires, and catheters are stocked in the special procedure area.

Direct Puncture Tray

2 Medicine glasses
1 Sponge forceps
4 Sterile towels
4 Towel clips
6 Sponges, 4″ x 4″
2 10 cc syringes
1 50 cc syringe
1 Knife blade, #11

NOTES

INDEX

A

B

C

M

N

O

P

R

S

T

V

W

Y

Z

XRAY LIBRARY
ROBERT L. MEALS D.O.